# THE FOOT BOOK

## Relief for Overused, Abused & Ailing Feet

### Glenn Copeland, D.P.M.
### with Stan Solomon

John Wiley & Sons, Inc.

New York • Chichester • Brisbane • Toronto • Singapore

*To Ruthie, my bride of eighteen years, and to the memory of my father-in-law, Aaron Tovye Zoladek, who became a very dear friend and advisor.*

Copyright © 1991, 1992 by Glenn Copeland and Stan Solomon Enterprises, Inc.

Published in Canada by Key Porter Books
Published in the United States by John Wiley & Sons, Inc.

This publication is provided to serve the reader as a supplement to professional medical guidance and treatment, and not as a substitute for professional medical care. As new medical research broadens our knowledge, changes in treatment and drug therapy are required. The author and publisher have made every effort to ensure that information regarding medical treatment is accurate and in accordance with the standards accepted at the time of publication. Readers are advised, however, to follow the product information sheet included with any drug administered and to seek professional advice before proceeding with medical treatment.

**Library of Congress Cataloging-in-Publication Data**
Copeland, Glenn.
    The foot book : relief for overused, abused & ailing feet / by
Glenn Copeland.
        p.     cm.
    Includes index.
    ISBN 0-471-55840-0 (pbk. : acid-free paper)
    1. Foot—Care and hygiene.   I. Title.
RD563.C668   1991
617.5′85—dc20                                                    91-43125

Printed in the United States of America
10 9 8 7 6 5 4 3
Printed and bound by Courier Companies, Inc.

# Contents

# Foreword

In the years since I wrote the foreword for *The Foot Doctor,* Glenn Copeland and I have continued to practice together while pursuing separate paths towards our common goal, the well-informed patient. Glenn and I have worked together since he joined the staff of Women's College Hospital in Toronto during the mid-1970s. Glenn has been available, and more than willing, to share his insight and clinical experience at the hospital's Lower Limb Clinic and as a podiatric consultant to the Canadian Back Institute. My surgical residents are often surprised to discover that several of the operative procedures I use in foot surgery are podiatric procedures I learned from Glenn Copeland. At present, Glenn and I are involved in research to further ascertain the relationship between low back pain and biomechanical foot disorders. As usual, I am cast in the role of skeptic. Although Glenn and I may disagree on our evaluation of problems, I have come to appreciate his belief that many complaints about low back pain can be traced to common foot faults. Hopefully our present study, which involves the use of computer-designed foot supports, will improve our understanding and even our level of agreement.

As an orthopedic surgeon, I am trained to identify a medical cause for a patient's complaint. As a podiatrist, Glenn Copeland is more apt to examine the way the patient walks. By combining our different points of view, we are often better able to evaluate a patient's problem and to provide an appropriate treatment program. All of us—Glenn, our patients and I— have benefited from our years of cooperation.

In his first book, Glenn Copeland dispelled many myths about foot care, and explained in simple language the causes of and treatments for the most common foot ailments. In *The Foot Book,* Glenn has updated and presented this information in separate sections for groups with special foot-care needs—pregnant women, patients with varicose veins, seniors, those involved in strenuous physical activities, and those with systemic disorders that affect the feet.

I value Glenn Copeland's podiatric opinions. This book gives you the opportunity to share his knowledge. It is a valuable addition to the growing list of health care books written for the non-medical reader.

Hamilton Hall, M.D., F.R.C.S.C.

# ACKNOWLEDGMENTS

This book could not have been written without the help, knowledge, and friendship of many people, all of whom deserve special mention.

I am indebted to my good friend, Theodore Ross, M.D., F.R.C.S.C., Department of Surgery, University of Toronto, who agreed to edit the chapter on varicose veins. Robbie Wolfe, M.D., F.R.C.P.C., cardiologist, Department of Medicine, University of Toronto, provided valuable advice for the medical chapters. His friendship and care over the past few years have been invaluable. Carol-Ann Reed, M.D., F.R.C.S.C., Department of Surgery, University of Toronto, has been a friend and mentor ever since I joined Women's College Hospital in 1977. Hamilton Hall, M.D., F.R.C.S.C., Department of Surgery, University of Toronto, is a special friend and office partner. His guidance and desire to share his expertise with me have been greatly appreciated. Jack Barkin, M.D., F.R.C.S.C., Department of Surgery (Urology), University of Toronto, has been one of my closest companions for many years. Ron Taylor, M.D. gave me the opportunity ten years ago to work with him at the S.C. Cooper Sports Medicine Clinic, Mount Sinai Hospital. He also enabled me to fulfil a dream when he asked me to become a podiatric consultant to the Toronto Blue Jays. Allan Gross, M.D., F.R.C.S.C., A.J. Latner Professor and Chairman, Division of Orthopaedic Surgery, University of Toronto, has allowed me to realize many of my career aspirations. I shall always treasure his unique sense of humor, and his willingness to share with me his medical endeavors.

I would also like to thank many members of the Toronto Blue Jays for extending to me the opportunity to be part of such a marvelous organization: Paul Beeston, Pat Gillick and Gord Ash in the front office; Tommie Craig, the trainer; Cito Gaston, the manager, who exemplifies the true meaning of teamwork; and Ernie Whitt and his wife Chris, who have shared many of the good and rocky times with me and my wife over the years, and who have taught us that every cloud does indeed have a silver lining.

My co-author, Stan Solomon, and his wife Linda Nagel have become close friends. How they ever survived another book with me is beyond my imagination. Thankfully, they did, because neither of my books would have been possible without Stan's efforts.

Finally, my family. My parents, Marg and Lou, and my brother, Marty, have always stood by me through thick and thin. My childhood sweetheart and loving wife, Ruthie, has shared all the wonderful times, and has stood by me through all the difficult years. Her love and devotion have made all the trials and tribulations worthwhile. And lastly, I thank my three children— Elyssa, Lauren and Aaron—who have brought so much love and joy into our lives.

G.C.

# 1.

# WHAT'S NEW, DOC?

SINCE I WROTE *THE FOOT DOCTOR* FIVE YEARS ago I have witnessed a profound increase in medical knowledge. And yet the lowly foot remains an overlooked, unglamorous appendage—the object of indifference to all but a handful of health care professionals. Foot ailments are rarely, if ever, life-threatening, so it is understandable that the medical profession gives short shrift to podiatric problems, even if they are often painful and debilitating. However, footwear manufacturers and the developers of medical diagnostic equipment have greatly contributed to the immense strides we have made in the past five years in the analysis and treatment of foot faults. Thanks to the introduction of sophisticated imaging techniques and computer read-outs, we are now in a much better position to provide our patients with an accurate early diagnosis and a treatment program to prevent more severe, long-term problems. Moreover, the recent advances in surgical techniques have often enabled us to treat those problems that require more radical intervention with a far greater degree of precision—and at much less discomfort to the patient—than was previously possible.

## Who Am I?

I believe that podiatrists are better able to diagnose and treat foot problems than others in the health care field. As a doctor of podiatric medicine, I am a qualified, registered practitioner licensed to treat conditions of the foot. Although legislation varies from district to district in North America, most states and provinces consider podiatrists primary-care practitioners. We are licensed to diagnose and treat—including surgically—conditions of and relating to the foot, even though we do not have an M.D. degree. When we graduate from one of the seven fully accredited colleges of podiatric medicine in the United States, we are given the designation of Doctor of Podiatric Medicine (D.P.M.). To get that far we must first obtain an undergraduate college or university education in either premedicine or one of the hard sciences.

One of the major differences between podiatrists and medical doctors is our advanced understanding of the biomechanics of the foot, as well as our training in ambulatory foot surgery. Biomechanics is the study of how the foot (and leg) function when the foot contacts the ground as a weight-bearing structure. Because I believe it to be the backbone of podiatric medicine, you will be reading a lot about biomechanics throughout this book.

## The Gaitway to Foot Care

In my opinion, the most significant advance in foot care in the past five years has been that of computerized gait analysis, which is a study of how we walk and run. Computerized gait analysis has, in part, confirmed our suspicions that abnormal walking patterns do indeed cause such maladies as bunions, hammer toes, neuromas (pinched nerves), and heel spurs. It has also taught us a great deal about why this is so, thereby helping us develop more effective treatment programs. Moreover, we are now better able to establish the relationship between foot abnormalities and  dysfunctions in other parts of the body, from the lumbar area of the back down to the lower leg.  I will have more to say about computer gait analysis in Chapter Two and about the relationship between the foot and physical problems elsewhere in the body in Chapter Seven. But before I continue, a case history of one of my patients will illustrate just how a foot dysfunction can create misery in another part of the anatomy. (There are many case histories in this book, most of them in the words of my patients, who are much more adept at describing their symptoms than I. At their request I have eliminated or changed their names to preserve their anonymity.)

A few months ago I was asked to examine the feet of a woman who had traveled to Canada from a country where podiatric medicine does not exist. This woman had been suffering for quite a few years from debilitating low back pain, which had not responded to any form of treatment in her homeland. When she arrived in Canada, she was examined by two prominent physicians. Both doctors concluded, independently, that she had terrible foot problems, which they believed to be responsible for her pain, and referred her to me.

When the woman arrived in my office her face was etched in pain. I took down her history with the help of her interpreter and examined her feet. They were truly a mess. I then had her walk across my computer gait analyzer, which clearly indicated severe biomechanical dysfunction in both feet. After explaining to her the significance of the computer print-out, I placed a pair of non-custom- made inserts into her shoes. I then asked her to take a walk up and down the halls for ten minutes.

Her initial reaction was one of amazement, followed by a broad grin. She burst out in her native language that her back felt better immediately—for the first time in years she was walking almost without pain. I told her to keep the inserts, but advised her to order the custom-made orthotics that would be based on her computer print-out. She agreed without a moment's hesitation.

The woman returned to my office two days later for a follow-up visit. I was curious to learn if the inserts had provided her with lasting relief, and was delighted to see her smiling. Her back pain had almost completely disappeared. I am convinced that faulty biomechanics was the primary cause of this woman's discomfort. She is a perfect example of the relationship between feet and other parts of the body, although her miraculous, instant relief is, alas, not quite the norm.

The complaints of my foreign patient are echoed by many athletes, most commonly runners, who are handicapped by an abnormal gait. This abnormality, which remains the most common cause of foot problems, is called pronation. It will be discussed repeatedly in the following chapters.

## New Surgical Techniques

Two trends have emerged in the past few years in podiatric practices across North America. Firstly, people who succumbed to footwear fashions of recent decades are now paying the price for their folly. Beatle boots, go-go boots, negative heeled shoes, and five-inch spiked heels have left their distorted marks on many feet. Disorders such as hammer toes and misaligned metatarsal bones are common occurrences for these unfortunate individuals.

Many of these conditions require surgery, and that is where the second trend becomes evident. We are living in an era of the "quick fix." Most of my patients argue that they don't have time to spend in hospitals or at home recuperating. If they require a surgical procedure, they want ambulatory care—that is, they want it to be over and done with fast, and in such a way that they can walk out of my office unaided and pain-free when the operation is finished. They hear about professional athletes who have arthroscopic knee surgery one day and are playing full tilt the next, and they think, "Why not me too?" Well, as you will see in Chapter Three, there aren't as many instant surgical fixes as you might think.

This is not to say that podiatric medicine has remained in the dark ages. It was only a few years ago that ingrown toenail surgery would bring the bravest, toughest athletes to tears and keep them in agony for hours, if not days. The procedure is now almost pain-free and involves little suffering afterwards. Moreover, the offending nail should never become ingrown again.

Aside from surgical procedures for ingrown nails, other foot surgery can now be done on an out-patient basis in the doctor's office. This includes surgery on hammer toes, other nail disorders, warts, minor bunions, neuromas, and metatarsal bones. The patients can walk out under their own power and recuperate quickly at home. A few years ago I operated on a bunionette (involving the baby toe) of one patient. At the same time I removed a growth from the bottom of her other foot. Despite my suggestion that she take the rest of the day off, she returned to her office immediately after the surgery and did not miss a single minute of work more than she had to.

Newspapers, tabloids, and periodicals are constantly writing about new miracle drugs, cures, diets, and surgical techniques. One of the hottest topics is laser surgery, which is being touted as the wonder treatment for anything from ingrown toenails to foot-and-mouth disease. From head to toe, lasers seem to be the way to go.

Despite their amazing uses and successes, lasers have not always proved to be as medically useful as was first thought, as you will learn in Chapter Three. Unfortunately, there are as many myths about laser surgery in the media as there are about Elvis being alive. Although medical practitioners initially hoped that laser beams might excise every known ailment, their disappointment to date has paralleled that of minimal-incision surgery. This technique, which involves tiny incisions to correct or remove a medical problem, is wonderfully effective for treating many disorders, but not all. Americans, in particular, who read newspaper advertisements about the efficacy of minimal-incision and laser surgical techniques to treat foot disorders would be wise to seek expert opinions before being exposed to the knife or the laser beam. I have great faith in lasers and minimal-incision surgery techniques, but they cannot cure every known malady.

## A Non-sexist Look at Women's Feet

Some of my female patients say that women deserve a chapter of their own in this book. I could not agree more. Most fashion shoes for women are still consistently ill fitting, although tremendous strides have been made in the past couple of years in women's athletic footwear. Pregnant women often maintain a busy work and social schedule almost to full term, so they must pay special attention to footwear to relieve discomforts often associated with pregnancy. I address this and other footwear problems specific to women in Chapter Four.

## What's "In," Doc?

A trend that began in the hippie days of the 1960s was to put comfort before style. Of course, "comfort" often became "style." In Southern California, where "cool" had nothing to do with the weather, tracksuits and running shoes were often *de rigueur* at informal functions. This fashion statement eventually spread across North America and has remained in vogue with a few designers and consumers who value comfort above all. Although many so-called yuppies have put their hippie days behind them, a new group of "California dreamers" appears to be emerging. Does this mean that non-supportive sandals and negative heels will make a big comeback? I hope that reason will prevail and that consumers will reject the absurd along with ridiculously high heels and pointed toes.

The word "wellness" became fairly common during the 1970s and is still with us. The goal of wellness is espoused by people who strive to "feel well" rather than merely to avoid disease.

In an attempt to fuel and feed off this sustained desire for personal comfort and well-being, athletic shoe manufacturers decided more than a decade ago to rethink sales strategy, with the emphasis on biomechanically sound, comfortable footwear. For those of us who had long preached the virtues of proper footwear to prevent foot and leg disorders, this was a significant breakthrough. What I do find absolutely astounding is that approximately 90 per cent of the athletic shoes bought today in North America are purchased by non-runners. This means that an ever-increasing number of people are regularly wearing shoes designed to help them prevent foot disorders rather than shoes that cause foot problems.

As you will learn in Chapter Six, many converts who have switched to running and walking shoes are seniors, who are learning that they can get the required amount of exercise without experiencing accompanying aches and pains.

### A Sporting Chance

Because of the initial fillip given by runners, one area of podiatry that has mushroomed in the past few years is that of sports medicine. Thanks to our new diagnostic equipment, we have now learned why and how changing the way a runner's foot strikes the ground—by placing an insert in his shoe—often dramatically relieves his discomfort. Although experts could previously explain this phenomenon as a correction of abnormal foot biomechanics, little was actually understood until recently about how such problems occurred. Therefore, treatment for the condition was not always completely effective, and specially designed shoes often exacerbated rather than relieved a problem. Those poorly designed shoes resulted in even worse biomechanics, which caused a wide range of disorders. I shall discuss footwear in detail in Chapter Eight.

We know now that if you change the angle of the foot, or the height of the heel, as it strikes the ground, you alter the gait pattern. We began to realize that some types of intervention to alter a person's gait did slow down or prevent wear-and-tear changes to parts of the body from the lower back to the big toe. We have now become quite adept at fine-tuning the biomechanics of a person's walking or running stride, in much the same way as contact lenses or glasses correct faulty vision.

But just in case you think we are on the threshold of podiatric nirvana, guess again. Trends change and novel ideas always produce new problems. We have a whole new range of overuse-related foot and leg injuries to combat (which will be discussed in Chapter Seven). Moreover, people are demanding alternative approaches to the treatment of sports injuries. "Locker-room" doctors dispensing anti-inflammatory and analgesic pills to fellow athletes have all but disappeared. Modern athletes are very concerned about the side effects of medications and are more reluctant to take them. The "no pain, no gain" philosophy of getting fit and treating injuries has also been largely discarded. It had been very popular with marathon runners, a diminishing breed.

## System Malfunctions

Most foot maladies are caused by poor biomechanics, which in turn can create havoc elsewhere in the body. However, there are some systemic disorders that can affect the foot or are enhanced by foot problems.

Chapter Five is devoted to a discussion of varicose veins. This is one problem that can be exacerbated by improper footwear. Since I first wrote (briefly) about varicose veins I have been approached by many of my patients who suffer from the disorder and do not know how to find relief. They are often particularly confused about the surgical techniques available today to treat the malady. Chapter Five should give you a complete understanding of the causes and various treatments for this condition and help you make a rational decision as to how to deal with it.

Many other systemic disorders involve the foot. And the diagnosis and treatment of them has been greatly enhanced by medical advances in recent years. For example, if you are a diabetic and have suffered from inflamed nerves in your feet, you will want to read Chapter Nine to learn about this discomforting byproduct of diabetes. There are now also dramatic improvements in the treatment of circulatory problems in the lower limbs, and they will also be examined in detail in Chapter Nine, as will many other systemic disorders, including gout.This chapter, written in a question-and-answer format, should help resolve some of the issues that most concern people with such problems.

Knowledge in the world of medicine generally triples every eight years, perhaps even faster as we rush towards the twenty-first century. Rest assured then that this is not a mere rehashing of my first book. Although I may touch on some familiar topics, most of the information is new.

When I announced to a friend that I was about to write a new book, he said, "You mean there's more?" There really is more to write about. The advances in diagnostic equipment—particularly bone scanners and new computer analysis techniques—are worthy of more than just the one chapter they can be afforded in this book. Despite my enthusiasm for this new technology, I constantly remind myself of the words of one of my college professors. "History tells us that medicine is an art, not merely a science," he told his students. "After all, we say we are 'practicing' our profession. We have not perfected it."

When he discussed modern diagnostic tools available to the medical practitioner, the professor stressed that we should never allow machines to replace what we have already learned from our studies and experiences. "We must use our acquired knowledge to properly interpret what the diagnostic tests are attempting to tell us. But we must make our diagnosis first. Otherwise we shall end up treating film and paper instead of the patient."

I like to think that I have acquired the knowledge to enable me to understand the information being divulged by the sophisticated equipment. I also think that it is important for you, the consumer of medical care, to have enough of this information at your disposal when you must make choices regarding the care of your feet. I trust that the information in the following chapters will enable you to make the right decisions.

# 2.

# SPACE-AGE DIAGNOSES

MEDICINE HAS TRULY EXCELLED IN THE PAST FEW years in its ability to look non-invasively inside the body. Until the development of scanners, magnetic resonance imagers, and ultrasound, doctors were forced to diagnose injury and disease by relying on an analysis of the symptoms and laboratory tests, an observation and evaluation of the patient's complaints, and, as a last resort, an invasive procedure such as surgery to examine the site of the problem. X-rays are valuable, but only for a limited range of physical abnormalities. Lab work—such as blood tests, urinalysis, and bacteriological surveys— may be inconclusive. Exploratory surgery is not without

13

its risks and discomforts, and is very costly. Occasionally, by the time a correct diagnosis of a disease or injury is made, it is either too late for effective treatment or the patient's recovery has been set back by the lack of, or improper, care.

However, we can now look forward to the day when quick, accurate diagnoses of injuries and diseases will become the norm rather than the exception. Imaging of the heretofore hidden parts of the body is now allowing medical professionals to distinguish definitively between normal and abnormal. It can often expose a myriad of varying internal conditions that we knew existed but were unable to see without complicated surgical techniques. Those of you who have seen the ultrasound imaging of a fetus in the womb, or watched your own heart beat, are aware of just how far medical science has advanced in recent years.

### New Scanning Techniques

Perhaps the most significant and talked-about development in the 1970s was the invention of the CAT (computerized axial tomography) scan. It allowed us to slice non-surgically through the body at different levels. It then took these various images and transformed them into one composite, comprehensive picture of the part of the body being photographed. This was our first non-invasive peek inside a vast area of the body. Since then different scanning techniques have helped tremendously in the diagnosis of numerous ailments, including specific foot problems. However, foot scans are hardly routine (except for emergencies), because of the cost of the procedure and the lack of quick availability of the scanners in most areas.

Scans can now pinpoint and diagnose conditions much earlier than before. For many injuries and diseases, this is the difference between life and death, or between quick, correct treatment and improper care.

Many different types of sophisticated scanners are now being used in medical diagnosis, developed to detect specific conditions in various parts of the body. Without getting into a complicated, detailed description, let me briefly describe how they work.

Patients either ingest or are injected with relatively harmless radioactive isotopes, substances that emit radiation and are attracted to certain body tissues. For example, gallium has an affinity for white blood cells, which attack infections in the body in order to destroy them. If a patient is suspected of having a bone infection (for example, osteomyelitis), which is not easy to detect using less sophisticated diagnostic tools, a bone (gallium 67-citrate) scan is done. The scan will pick up and measure high gallium emissions from the site of the disorder, because there will be an unusual number of white cells fighting the infection. Before the development of such scans, a bone infection was difficult to detect until a regular x-ray showed the moth-eaten appearance of the bone, which was caused by damage inflicted by the bacteria.

Another type of scan that is particularly useful involves the use of thallium, which is absorbed by cardiac muscle tissue. Thallium scans are a marvelously effective way of detecting arterial blockages that affect the heart muscle. Although these scans are not the sole method used to determine the damage caused by and treatment for such blockages, they can replace more invasive diagnostic procedures when the condition is initially being assessed.

The bone scan, which employs another radioactive isotope to discover stress fractures that regular x-rays are unable to pick up, is often used to diagnose foot problems. X-rays routinely read fractures when bone has been displaced, but cannot usually show stress fractures of a bone that has not been badly broken or displaced. The particular  isotope used in this case, technetium-methylene-diphosphonate, is greatly attracted to osteoblasts, cells that are responsible for the growth and repair of bones.

Why are we interested in examining the foot to locate possible increased osteoblastic activity? Often I see patients who have suffered some sort of trauma to a foot; sometimes the injury is due primarily to overstress, which makes diagnosis difficult because the cause cannot be pinpointed immediately. The symptoms may be significant swelling in the affected area and pain to the touch. The x-ray is negative but inconclusive, because it rarely picks up stress fractures—particularly of the tiny bones in the feet.

Before bone scans were developed I could only guess that the problem was a stress fracture and treat the patient accordingly, and then wait six to eight weeks for the next x-ray to show, I hoped, the natural bone-healing process. Or I could diagnose the problem as some other condition, and perhaps prescribe the wrong type of therapy. Now the bone scans can verify the diagnosis of a fracture by indicating the abnormal number of osteoblasts present where the break occurred. Proper treatment can be begun immediately, and the patient can be reassured that the diagnosis is correct, thereby being spared a great deal of anxiety.

## The Ultra Diagnostic Tool

When medical professionals realized that regular x-rays might be unsafe for expectant mothers and unborn children, they had to find an alternative way of determining the status of the pregnancy, particularly when problems might be expected. It was discovered that ultrahigh sound waves could be passed harmlessly into the body, rebound back to the probe, and be translated into a picture on a monitor.

In podiatry we use ultrasound diagnostic procedures more for soft-tissue evaluation than for bone abnormalities. It is particularly useful for identifying foreign objects buried in the foot—a real problem for people who have a habit of walking barefoot in places littered with damaging bits of debris. It has also recently been proved that ultrasound can be particularly useful in discovering bone fractures of the foot, especially in the sesamoid bones, fractures that are often quite difficult to detect (see Diagram 1).

Another development is the possible use of ultrasonography to diagnose neuromas in the foot. These pinched nerves can be quite difficult to detect and may be confused with other foot problems that might require different treatment. It has recently been shown that ultrasound can show an area of thickening around the inflamed nerve, which would help indicate the presence of a neuroma.

Because ultrasound diagnostic equipment and maintenance is inexpensive compared with other sophisticated procedures, I expect further exciting developments in its use, including the detection of foot disorders. Whenever possible, I would prefer to use

*Diagram 1*
**Bones of the Foot**

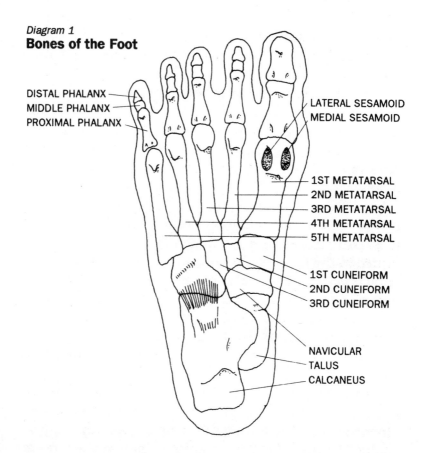

DISTAL PHALANX
MIDDLE PHALANX
PROXIMAL PHALANX

LATERAL SESAMOID
MEDIAL SESAMOID

1ST METATARSAL
2ND METATARSAL
3RD METATARSAL
4TH METATARSAL
5TH METATARSAL

1ST CUNEIFORM
2ND CUNEIFORM
3RD CUNEIFORM

NAVICULAR
TALUS
CALCANEUS

ultrasonic diagnostic equipment instead of scans to diagnose tricky foot conditions because there would be no potential radiation exposure or disposal problems to deal with.

## The New Kid on the Block

No medical facility should be without a magnetic resonance imager (MRI), the latest, most accurate way of non-invasively examining the inside of the body. Unfortunately, the prohibitive costs of buying and setting up MRIs prevent most facilities from owning one. This is particularly true in Canada, where it is difficult for politicians to rationalize the initial expense of the imager when the government-funded health care services are already hard-pressed to meet existing minimal demands. In Toronto, Canada's largest city, only two MRIs are in operation as I write. Contrast this with a city like Los Angeles, where many hospitals have eagerly paid large sums to have this ultimate diagnostic tool at their disposal.

The beauty of the MRI is its amazing ability to differentiate precisely the normal from the abnormal and one type of tissue from another. It is even more accurate than CAT scanning, and does not require the use of radioactive materials. The patient does not usually have to ingest or be injected with anything; he or she is scanned in a magnetic field, and the resulting images are recorded and shown on a monitor. Therefore, it appears to be a very safe diagnostic tool.

The value of MRIs is most apparent in their ability to provide medical experts with vital information when they are examining the brain and spinal column. For example, the imagers clearly show herniated spinal discs or stenosis (narrowing) of the spinal canal, even more precisely than CAT scanners do. And where they are available they could replace the use of the invasive, painful myelogram, which surgeons have employed for years as their atlas of the spine.

MRIs can often provide early identification of medical problems and guide the treatment process, so that proper care with minimal, if any, in-patient care can be quickly undertaken. In the long run this breakthrough in diagnostic equipment could result in dramatic savings to the medical consumer and governments, and, of course, save lives.

Because foot problems are rarely life-threatening, and in view of the present costs and demands on the usage of MRIs, it is unlikely that podiatrists will soon be able to enjoy ready access to these imagers. It's a pity, because I have seen just how clearly an MRI was able to pick up a fracture of a sesamoid bone. However, one of these days MRIs will be affordable for most medical practitioners, and will come in various sizes and shapes, so that even podiatrists will find it possible and convenient to install them in their offices. In any event, MRIs are the wave of the future, and may conceivably make obsolete other types of non-invasive investigations of the body that rely on radiation.

### A Computer Mega-step

Computerized gait analysis is a major improvement in the understanding and accurate diagnosis of foot abnormalities that can create many painful disorders of the lower limbs. Specialized computers can now precisely measure poor foot mechanics and have made it possible for us to understand how a great many of these lower limb and spinal problems are created. Moreover, the initial cost of the diagnostic equipment is not earth-shattering, although it does involve some sophisticated computer hardware and software.

Biomechanics is the study of the way people walk and run. When we analyze their biomechanics we are trying to evaluate how the body weight is distributed on the feet as they come in contact with the ground and continue through the weight-bearing phase of the stride. We have long been able to record on film the way people walk, run, and play. However, interpretation has been difficult, because data collection has been based strictly on observation. This has all changed.

The importance of the biomechanics of the human gait was acknowledged as far back as Roman times. It gained new respect in the last century in parts of Asia and Europe, where people with foot pain were often treated with arch supports. In the early 1900s downhill skiers began to realize that they could ski more quickly and comfortably by "canting" their boots—raising one side of the boot—to try to even out their center of gravity as they raced down the slopes. Their unscientific analysis proved to be well grounded: most serious downhill skiers have been wearing special inserts in their ski boots for years, with excellent results in comfort and performance.

Eventually this empirical trial-and-error approach to proper foot mechanics led to intensive scientific research. It has culminated in the past five years in a sophisticated analysis of the relationships between the biomechanics of parts of the foot, the lower back, hip, knee, and leg. This exciting development, enhanced by the introduction of high-tech video cameras, high-resolution monitors, electronic treadmills, and special computer equipment, has enabled us to confirm many of the theories we have long espoused.

When I first wrote about foot disorders, most evaluations of a person's gait were done "statically": the patient remained seated while measurements were made of certain angles of the foot and a cast was created. Although we could learn much by watching people walk and run, it was nearly impossible to quantify or evaluate the hundreds of motions occurring in the lower leg and foot, the effects on weight-bearing parts of the foot, and their interactions. Yet as I learned more about the relationships among the various bones from the hips to the knees and down to the feet, I realized that it was vitally important to become more encompassing in my observations. I was no longer concentrating strictly on watching the foot when it struck the ground and carried through to the lift-off motion. Since natural walking movements are quite rapid, and because of the increasing availability of sophisticated video cameras, it was logical to develop stop-action video analysis as a useful tool. Not only could athletes have their movements analyzed to maximize their effectiveness and efficiency but podiatrists could use the technique to "compartmentalize" and evaluate a person's gait to determine whether a fault existed.

Although stop-action videos were a major achievement, the technique still failed to provide a definitive analysis of what happened to the bottom of the foot when it hit the ground and continued through to lift-off. Moreover, it failed to reveal precisely how weight was transferred from one part of the foot to another. The normal foot pronates just the right amount when it comes in contact with the ground—that is, the weight is initially borne by the outside of the foot and is then evenly distributed in a rolling motion across the forefoot until near the end of the step. As the body weight reaches the area of the big toe joint in the normal walking or running gait, the opposite of pronation—supination—occurs. At this point—the propulsive stage of the gait—the rolling motion to the big toe is stopped as the heel is lifted off the ground. In abnormal pronation, the normal pronation rolling motion is exaggerated and continues to the big toe side of the foot. People with this abnormality tend to strike the ground on the outside part of the heel and end up rolling excessively across the forefoot. As a result the big toe joint often winds up bearing too much of the weight, which ought to be evenly distributed among it and the second and third toe joints. Poor weight distribution of this type  was causing a host of foot, leg, knee, hip, and lower back disorders among a large number of the runners podiatrists and orthopods began to treat in the 1970s and 1980s.

It was fairly simple for the trained eye to recognize pronation by watching a person walk. But I was constantly troubled by our inability to measure accurately the degree of pronation. I was also concerned about not being able to pinpoint the exact way a person pronated.  For example, when the foot hit the ground, did most of the pronation occur in the rearfoot or the forefoot? Did both parts of the foot pronate, and was it equal? If the rearfoot was the cause of pronation, what did the forefoot do to try to compensate for the abnormality, and vice versa? It became obvious to me that some sort of computerized gait analysis of every fraction of the bottom of the foot was essential to answer these questions. I wanted to be able to measure precisely the order in which parts of the foot struck the ground in the gait cycle, and the exact amount of weight placed on each square millimeter when it was in contact with the ground. To that end I began to look for the ultimate measuring device.

Five years ago I was experimenting with an apparatus that had eight to ten sensors that could be attached to various spots on the bottom of the foot. The sensors would provide weight-bearing measurements, but only for those parts of the foot to which they were attached. I was intrigued by the approach but dissatisfied with the results, and I began a search for a sophisticated computer package that would provide weight-bearing measurements for the entire foot. For the past three years I have been intimately involved in the development of such a diagnostic device with a computer firm specializing in medical applications for their products. I can report that the equipment I am now using can provide me with those precise measurements I require to analyze and treat a foot disorder caused by poor biomechanics. In the next couple of years I expect to be able to use more advanced computer software to read and analyze the measurements of all my patients. In this way we shall be in a position to discern patterns of all common foot conditions, to confirm precisely what is normal and abnormal, and even predict problems when no symptoms yet exist. The prospects are very exciting!

What does all this mean to the person with a foot problem? I am a strong believer in shoe inserts—orthotics—to correct biomechanical faults. By being able to analyze with finite precision the degree of the problem and the part or parts of the foot causing it, we can now prescribe orthotics that are much more likely to correct the fault than previously, when we relied on static measurements—castings and foam impressions of the foot, which were made while the patient was not moving. Now the patient walks barefoot across a plate that transfers the information to the computer, which produces a print-out that provides a precise measurement of how the weight has been distributed on each square millimeter of the foot. This print-out provides the orthotics manufacturer with all the information needed to produce an insert that provides the exact weight-bearing corrections the patient requires to correct his or her imperfect biomechanics. (See Chapter Eight for a detailed discussion of orthotics.)

How do we know that our patients have been properly diagnosed and treated? First of all we have their own, albeit subjective, comments. The overwhelming majority of our patients who have been analyzed by our computerized equipment report that their problems have all but disappeared after wearing their new orthotics for a few weeks. Secondly, we have the objective read-outs of the impersonal computer. We have our patients wear their new orthotics for three weeks before returning to our office for an evaluation. When we put them on the machine—in their shoes with the orthotics inserted—the print-outs invariably show that the unequal weight distribution that caused their problems has been corrected.

Aside from the dramatic relief my patients experience after computerized gait analysis and treatment with proper inserts, there is another major bonus for me. I have now begun to learn just why many foot abnormalities and deformities develop. For example, bunions and other big toe disorders are caused by excessive pronation during the "toe-off" phase of the gait, when the foot is about to leave the ground and is pushing off. Before computer gait analysis we never really understood the dynamics that cause these disorders. Now we know that abnormal retroactive forces (when the big toe is forced backwards) cause the big toe joint to become deformed or unduly stressed. So, we have to concentrate on controlling weight distribution better on that part of the foot once the weight has left the metatarsus. Before computerized gait analysis we did not know precisely where the weight was distributed after it left the metatarsus. Now we have the exact answer, and we can more accurately correct the problem.

I don't expect every podiatrist in North America to have computerized gait analysis equipment in his or her office. Neither do I argue that all foot problems can be accurately diagnosed and treated just with the use of this equipment. Yet podiatry has entered the space age with sophisticated diagnostic and therapeutic equipment, and people need no longer resign themselves to a lifetime of aching feet. However, as you will see in the following chapters, solutions to foot problems do not reside totally in the domain of the computer.

# 3

# CONSUMER-
# FRIENDLY FOOT
# CARE

IN THIS CHAPTER I WILL CONCENTRATE ON THE
treatment of foot disorders that are primarily a result of
poor biomechanics—bunions, hammer toes, corns, and
calluses. I shall also deal with plantar warts, which are
caused by a virus, and other maladies not directly
associated with biomechanical problems. But first, a word
about surgery.

Space-age technology is not only threatening to make
invasive diagnostic procedures obsolete, it is also affecting
the treatment end of medical care. For centuries the word
"surgery" has struck fear into the hearts of patients faced
with some form of invasive treatment procedure. In the

not-too-distant future it will provoke excitement and intrigue rather than alarm.

When it comes to foot surgery, major advances in invasive corrective techniques could not have happened too soon. One problem of conventional foot or leg surgery—unlike operations on other parts of the body—is that people must be able to bear weight comfortably on the limb afterwards in order to get around. Crutches, canes, walkers, or other appliances cannot be considered a long-term or permanent solution. If surgery leaves patients with an area of painful scar tissue on the bottom of the foot, how will they be able to walk normally again? Also, older surgical techniques to correct bony deformities in the lower limbs often fail to eliminate the abnormal biomechanics that caused the problem.

Surgical techniques have not changed dramatically in the past five years, although they have vastly improved. Significant progress has been made in treating podiatric conditions by combining refined surgical techniques with follow-up orthotic measures to help prevent recurrence of the disorder. Also, because of our ability now to diagnose foot problems more accurately, we are more likely to be successful when we are forced to operate to cure the condition.

### Front-end Alignment

Many myths still circulate about how bunions develop. A bunion (hallux valgus) is basically a deviation in the joint of the big toe (see Diagram 2). The affected big toe with the tell-tale bump looks unsightly and is painful when irritated by shoes that cannot conform to the shape of the protrusion. But shoes are not the cause of the bunion, although they can obviously exacerbate the discomfort if they are tight-fitting. Bunions are caused by abnormal biomechanics, not vice versa as was once thought. Over-pronation is the culprit, and it may be aided by a hereditary predisposition—the structure of the foot a person inherited. One of my patients is a young woman who has begun to develop bunions on both feet. Both of her parents have had foot problems, and her mother had bunion surgery a few years ago. The young woman has opted to wear orthotics in the hope that her bunions will not become unmanageable.

If abnormal pronation is identified and corrected early enough with properly prescribed orthotic devices, the formation of a bunion can be prevented. However, if the bunion has already developed and cannot be tolerated by the patient, I would then opt for state-of-the-art surgery.

Textbooks on the surgical treatment of bunions first appeared more than a century ago. The techniques ranged from amputation of the affected toe to variations of treatments commonly used on hands. As we now know, these operations hardly cured the disorder. When the toe was left intact the bunion usually reappeared in the next few years, because the surgery failed to correct the causative biomechanical fault. Of course, amputation of the big toe only enhanced the patient's biomechanical abnormalities, and left him perpetually off-balance with a sad-looking foot.

Fortunately, amputation of the big toe ceased to be a treatment for bunions many generations ago, but the other techniques still failed adequately to correct the cause of the condition. Only in the past few years have surgical procedures been developed to incorporate the realignment of the bone with the correction of the abnormal

*Diagram 2*
**Formation of a Bunion**

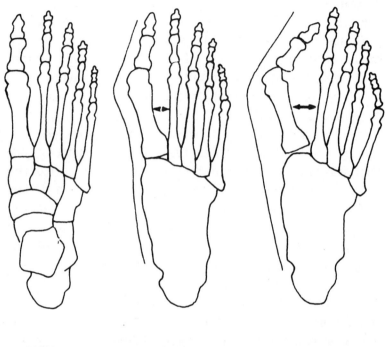

NORMAL                MILD                SEVERE

motion that led to the deformity.

As shown in Diagram 2, the first metatarsal bone and the bones of the big toe have been pulled out of alignment, forming a bunion. Until recently, surgery has been performed to realign these bones so that the bump disappears and the affected toe looks normal. Yet the abnormal pressure on the big toe remained, because the excess pronation had not been corrected. The first metatarsal bone was still being unduly stressed. As a result, it would eventually be pulled out of alignment again, and a new bunion would form. This development can be partially prevented if the person wears orthotics to balance properly the distribution of weight on the foot when it is in contact with the ground. However, one bone is still out of its proper position.

To overcome this problem, surgical techniques have been devised that not only move the wayward bones into proper alignment but also slide the first metatarsal downwards so that its head is pushed into a normal position. In its proper position the metatarsal bone can help prevent the over-pronation that caused the formation of the bunion. Combined with proper orthotic devices, this surgical breakthrough has provided very encouraging results. Once the patient has fully recovered from the surgery, we do a computerized gait analysis of his stride. The positive results so far augur well, and we believe that the new surgery plus the use of orthotics will almost completely prevent the recurrence of the bunion. There is another bonus. Previous surgical techniques often required a general anesthetic and a hospital stay of about one week, followed by a month or two of rest, during which the patient was required to wear a non-walking cast. Now, the procedure can usually be done on an out-patient basis under a local anesthetic, and the patient can leave almost immediately after.

Of course, we would like to be able to avoid entirely the need for bunion surgery and other types of foot surgery, but that is not always possible. However, if we isolate a biomechanical problem and treat it early enough with orthotic or orthopedic devices, we can often prevent the need for any future corrective surgery. Preventive care is now a reality, thanks to our recently acquired knowledge of the damage abnormal foot structures and poor biomechanics can wreak on the poor unsuspecting sole and other parts of the foot.

On the other hand, corrective surgery is occasionally necessary when an abnormality cannot otherwise be corrected. For example, a person who is bow-legged may require an operation to straighten out leg bones to prevent subsequent serious damage to bones and joints in the lower extremities, damage that can be permanent or repaired only by more complicated, comprehensive surgery. A typical example of this approach when the feet are involved is minor surgery to correct a hammer toe.

## The Hammer Woe

Hammer toes are caused by a biomechanical fault that involves a dropped metatarsal head and abnormally tight tendons in the affected toe (see Diagram 3). If you bend your middle finger at the knuckle, you will approximate the appearance of a hammer toe. What characterizes this condition is the growth of hard tissue—a corn—atop the raised part of the toe. The corn is nature's way of protecting the bones and joint from irritation that is produced by the tops of shoes.

Before the development of computerized gait analysis we knew that a patient with a hammer toe was subjected to undue stress on that toe, but we did not know precisely how and where the problem occurred. Now we can tell exactly why the toe is being bent out of shape. Using the computer print-out of the weight-bearing distribution on

*Diagram 3*
## A Hammer Toe and the Extensor and Flexor Tendons

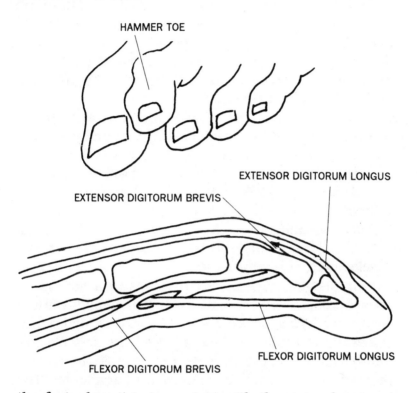

HAMMER TOE

EXTENSOR DIGITORUM LONGUS

EXTENSOR DIGITORUM BREVIS

FLEXOR DIGITORUM LONGUS

FLEXOR DIGITORUM BREVIS

the foot when it is in contact with the ground, we can design orthotics to alleviate the imbalance. If the patient still complains of a painful toe, and if the bones in the affected toe have yet to be damaged, we will do what is called a soft-tissue release.

When the head of the metatarsal bone drops, the tendons in the affected toe tighten, which causes the joint in the toe to push upwards. If a person with a hammer toe were to go barefoot all the time, a hammer toe would not likely pose a problem. However, when, for example, a woman with a hammer toe fits her foot into a high-heeled shoe with a tiny toe-box, the raised toe joint begins to rub against the shoe. To avoid an inflammation of the offended site, hard tissue develops atop the skin to protect the joint. This is a typical hard corn. Unfortunately, there are very sensitive nerve endings under the corn, so the area eventually begins to hurt terribly whenever it is irritated. Finally, the woman has trouble fitting into any normal type of footwear and seeks medical help. She may be lucky enough to find relief solely with the use of orthotics and trimming of the corn. If not, the next step will be soft-tissue release surgery, followed by the continued wearing of orthotics.

Before we understood that the abnormally positioned metatarsal head was primarily responsible for the development of hammer toes, surgery was confined to cutting (lengthening) affected tendons in a soft-tissue release procedure. When tendons are cut the ends will find each other during the healing process and reattach, which is why the procedure is often called lengthening. We now know that this procedure is not enough to correct permanently the condition causing the hammer toe. The head of the offending metatarsal bone must also be raised to a normal position; otherwise the hammer toe may eventually recur. This is done by having the patient wear orthotics. Computer gait analysis of a patient before combined surgery and orthotic treatment will clearly define the abnormality causing the hammer toe. If the patient has the hammer toe surgery but is not fitted with orthotics, subsequent gait analysis will show that the metatarsal head abnormality still exists. But when the person has the surgery and is then fitted with orthotics, computer gait analysis done when the healing process is complete indicates that the abnormality has been corrected.

The surgical techniques for treating hammer toes have changed little in recent years. Yet we now understand much better the dynamics involved in the development of this condition and can take preventive measures to ensure that the problem does not recur.

A few words of caution to those who believe that they can live with the discomfort of a hammer toe and who abhor the thought of visiting medical practitioners. Firstly, hammer toes and hard corns are not serious conditions—only painful. But people often consciously alter their gait to avoid pressure on the sore toes. As soon as they begin to walk or run abnormally, they are opening themselves up to a whole new range of lower limb problems. Secondly, the surgery, if required, can be done fairly quickly in the doctor's office under a local anesthetic. Patients can then look forward to a rapid recovery with minimal discomfort. So why suffer needlessly when the treatment is simple and benign?

## Kissing Corns

Soft corns are caused when toes are squeezed together by ill-fitting shoes, and by bones in the affected toes that are abnormally shaped and protrude against each other (see Diagram 4). The side of one toe lies tightly against an adjacent toe and the toe bone begins to jut out. A soft corn develops to protect the exposed bone from irritation. Occasionally the same thing happens to the adjacent toe and a corn also forms on it for the same reason. These

*Diagram 4*
**The Formation of a Soft Corn**

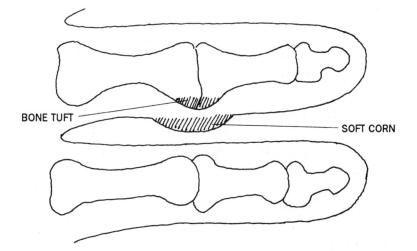

corns begin to rub together—hence the term "kissing corns"—and can cause extreme burning and stinging discomfort between the toes. The pain has been known to bring grown men to their knees.

When I first wrote about soft corns I prescribed very simple treatment for mild cases. I trimmed the corn and applied a donut pad to protect the area from further irritation. I also advised the patient to switch to better-fitting shoes. For those people who did not respond to non-invasive treatment I would perform a simple surgical procedure—an exostectomy—which involved shaving down the exposed part of the bone causing the problem. This procedure, which has been improved over the years with the development of better instrumentation, can be done in about twenty minutes in the doctor's office under a local anesthetic. There is almost no discomfort following the surgery; the patient may require at the most two stitches and a small adhesive bandage. Recovery time is quite rapid, and the patient can usually return to normal activities immediately after the operation, providing she does not attempt to run a marathon the same day.

However, soft corns can return unless the underlying problem is solved. Therefore, it is essential that preventive measures be taken—shoes that fit properly, and, if necessary, orthotics to correct any biomechanical problem that may have helped distort the toe.

### Callus Observations

Calluses are often thought of as corns on the bottom of the foot. Indeed they are nothing more than hard tissue that forms under a dropped metatarsal head (see Diagram 5). When the bone is out of alignment, it is subjected to excess stress when the foot is in contact with the ground.

The callus develops to protect the bone, which has been forced to accept an abnormal amount of weight. And, because nerve endings on the bottom of the feet are exquisitely sensitive and close to the surface, the pain can be quite excruciating for people who are on their feet for prolonged periods.

To give you an idea of just how painful calluses can be, let me quote the words of one of my patients, who, unfortunately, exacerbated her condition by attempting

*Diagram 5*
**A Dropped Metatarsal Head and
Formation of a Callus**

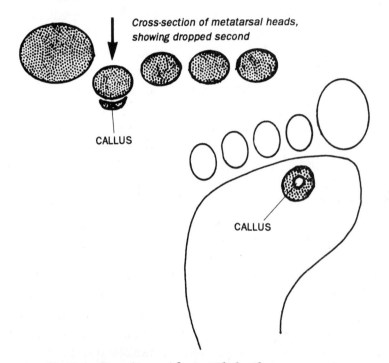

*Cross-section of metatarsal heads,
showing dropped second*

CALLUS

CALLUS

to alleviate her discomfort with bathroom surgery.

"The soles of both feet hurt, and I had very painful calluses. The worst part was when I had to get up in the morning. My feet would hurt so much that I could not walk at all for a few minutes when I got out of bed.I tried to remove the calluses with corn plasters, and wound up with holes in my feet where I had burned away a lot of good skin along with the calluses."

When this woman was referred to me by her family physician her feet were a mess. Fortunately, she responded well to orthotics and has not been troubled with calluses for several years. Because of the senior management position she holds, she is required to dress well, and wears fashion orthotics in all her shoes. She was recently in my office to get a new pair of graphite orthotics. As she was leaving she said, "Until people have been through this, they do not realize how much of an effect painful feet have on the way you feel about everything."

Computer gait analysis has revealed the presence of tremendous shearing forces, which occur in the foot where calluses form. Sometimes, calluses form under many or all the metatarsal heads, indicating a widespread weight-distribution problem. As with the disorders I have already discussed, the treatment for calluses depends on the severity of the situation and now includes preventive maintenance with orthotic devices.

Orthotics will often obviate the need for surgery to eliminate the causes of calluses. Thanks to the development of podiatric computer technology, the devices are much more likely to be successful today than they were five years ago. (I shall have much to say about orthotics in Chapter Eight.) But when the problem is acute and cannot be cured only by wearing orthotics, surgery may be necessary. However, there is one new technique that could be considered for patients who are poor surgical risks (for example, diabetics).

If only one of the metatarsal heads has dropped, the wearing of orthotics could be combined with an injection of medical-grade collagen into the area under the offending bone. Collagen is a primary component of connective tissue, bone, skin, and other soft tissues. It is injected under the skin by dermatologists and plastic surgeons to smooth out wrinkles. When injected through the top of the foot and down to the sole under the inflamed metatarsal head, it forms a solid, strong fat pad, which protects the bone from the hard surface below it. So, when a person is walking, he or she will have an extra cushion under the metatarsal bone to help absorb the weight. Therefore, the collagen eliminates the need for the development of a callus to protect the bone. Unfortunately, early studies have indicated that the injected collagen begins to break down after only a few months and, eventually, its beneficial effects diminish to near zero. At this point a second injection can be tried, or a surgical procedure can be done to help provide a permanent solution to the problem.

Metatarsal osteotomies—surgery to position and align properly an abnormal bone—are very effective in treating calluses that do not respond sufficiently to non-invasive orthotic measures. Once the metatarsal bones have been correctly positioned and weight is properly distributed across the forefoot when a person is walking, the calluses will disappear. They no longer need to develop to protect the head of the metatarsal. Obviously, though, weight distribution must remain normal or similar problems may occur, so orthotics should be worn after surgery to prevent such a recurrence.

### Minimalism

There is a major controversy among medical professionals about minimal-incision surgery versus open surgery. The difference between minimal-incision and open surgery techniques is night and day. The former technique relies more on the surgeon's feel; the latter, being a larger incision that completely exposes the area to be operated on, allows the surgeon to see precisely what he or she is doing. Minimal-incision instruments are smaller than those used in traditional methods of surgery.

The advantage of minimal-incision surgery is that there is much less cutting, at least on the surface. Therefore, fewer if any stitches or clamps are required and scarring is kept to a minimum. This is often an important consideration, particularly in foot surgery, because scar tissue can become quite painful when irritated. Surgery on any part of the foot—particularly the weight-bearing bottom—can leave scarring that may become inflamed by the constant rubbing of the shoe or when the foot is in contact with the ground. On the other hand, because the surgeon cannot see the entire area being operated on, the chances of error are greater. In the right hands, minimal-incision surgery can be very successful with minimal trauma to the affected area. In the wrong hands, it can lead to unpleasant complications.

Surgeons opposed to minimal-incision techniques are often practitioners who were trained only in the more traditional open surgery. They believe that what they cannot see may hurt you much more than a bit more scarring. They regularly question the training of minimal-incision surgeons and the results of their labors. This controversy has not changed in the past few years.

Unfortunately, I am aware of no scientific research that can conclusively prove the favorable or poor results of minimal-incision surgery. However, a few studies do indicate one definite trend. Good results from minimal-incision techniques usually go unnoticed; patients do not complain when their operation has been completely successful. When such surgery is botched, patients often wind up in the care of traditional surgeons, who will willingly share their opinion with the world that their way is still the best.

Foot doctors are not the only minimalists practicing medicine today. Minimal-incision surgery on backs and other parts of the body is regularly performed by neurosurgeons and orthopods, often with startling success. I strongly believe that such surgery scores the best marks when surgeons have been trained in both techniques. They should know instinctively which procedure best fits the criteria. If I were a medical consumer requiring foot care, I would think twice about choosing a podiatrist who claimed to be able to treat all operable conditions with minimal-incision surgery. The same applies to those who advertise laser treatments as a cure for all podiatric problems.

Today most soft corn surgery is done using minimal incision procedures. When other types of foot surgery are involved, I am guided by the amount of bone work involved. Many bunions can successfully be operated on using closed techniques; but, when the surgery is complicated, I would prefer to be able to see the field of action rather than rely strictly on feel. The same applies to hammer toes and metatarsal osteotomies. As one of my orthopedic colleagues, a proponent of open surgery, once noted, "The incision doesn't heal from end to end, but from side to side." What she was saying is that the size of the incision is not as important as a surgeon's technique and careful approach, which will reduce trauma just as easily as minimal-incision procedures. All surgical procedures produce trauma; bones are still broken and realigned, and soft tissue is still damaged.

## Star Wars Surgery

A day rarely passes in which I am not asked about or subjected to more information on lasers—Light Amplification by Stimulated Emission of Radiation. Lasers emit thin beams of light that release tremendous amounts of heat energy. They are now being used to zap eye cataracts, skin blemishes, and a host of other body abnormalities. At this time, lasers cannot cut through anything that is less than 70 per cent water. Since bones are less than 70 per cent water, lasers cannot be used for bone surgery, aside from making the initial incision through the soft tissue. So forget about laser bunion surgery for the present.

The jury is still out on the uses of lasers for podiatric purposes. Two podiatrists recently told me that they have discontinued laser surgery to remove plantar warts. The procedure is painful and can leave significant scarring on the bottom of the foot. You can imagine how it would feel constantly to bear weight on a large scar. Moreover, the success rate is not that high. In fact, the two podiatrists have enjoyed as much if not more success on plantar warts using liquid nitrogen.

The other common podiatric use for lasers is to remove ingrown nails. Once again, the results are not earth-shattering. The procedure can be more painful than the phenol-alcohol procedure I regularly use. I also believe that, unlike the latter technique, laser surgery might leave a few nail-growing cells intact, thereby allowing for the re-formation of an ingrown nail.

Because I do not use lasers for podiatric surgery, I have consulted with two of my colleagues who are experts in such procedures. Both feel very strongly that, although lasers have been over-advertised, they have dramatically reduced trauma and increased healing time in toenail surgery, wart removal, and soft-tissue surgery.

So, I remain of two minds. My advice to someone in search of foot care is to find a podiatric surgeon who is well versed in all aspects of podiatric surgery and who can explain fully the advantages and disadvantages of the various procedures.

### Feeling No Pain

One of the major advances in out-patient surgery has been the development of short- and long-term anesthetics. They can just about eliminate pain and alleviate the need for the patient to take analgesics or stronger drugs to relieve post-surgery discomfort. I recall telling one patient of a new local anesthetic I was about to use on him. He became quite agitated. "I don't want any of the local stuff, Doc," he said, frowning. "Get me the imported stuff." He must have thought I was about to give him a swig of home-made wine.

### Kids' Stuff

Finally, good news about children's feet. Some of the major advances in foot care in the last five years have occurred in the treatment of young feet that toe in or out, or legs that turn inwards or outwards. A number of orthopedic appliance manufacturers have developed devices that not only help straighten the lower limbs but also are more easily tolerated by children. These "counter-rotational" type devices are much easier to fit and adjust than previous types, and often do not require special footwear. Moreover, they may soon replace the use of casts, which are cumbersome and uncomfortable for children.

Any parent who suspects that an offspring has a lower leg or foot problem should have the child evaluated by a specialist in children's orthopedic or podiatric problems. By accurately diagnosing and treating such a problem early in the game, a host of future lower limb disorders can be avoided. I would compare the need to attack the problems early with that of orthodontia to correct children's dental dysfunctions. Wouldn't you want your children's legs and feet to be as straight as their teeth? With the modern devices that have been developed, there is no need for a child today to go without proper foot and leg care.

More on the subject of children. I alluded earlier to the role of heredity in the development of bunions. Well, many other biomechanical foot disorders can flare up in children of parents who have their own foot problems. It is not uncommon for me to see children with a variety of biomechanical faults that are quite similar to those of their parents. I can think of one family in particular, three of whom have been treated by me.

Mike was first seen by me in 1985. He had continuous pains in his lower legs and feet from both plantar fasciitis and Achilles tendinitis, which were caused by over-pronation. He has been wearing orthotics regularly since then, and his problems have disappeared.

In June 1990 Mike's wife appeared in my office. She was suffering from acute pain in the heel area, and had been told two years earlier by her doctor that she had heel spurs. Judging by her symptoms—acute pain when she first put weight on her foot in the morning and increased discomfort when she played tennis—it was obvious that she had also developed plantar fasciitis. I also prescribed orthotics for her, which she has not worn regularly. As a consequence, she still suffers significant discomfort.

One month later the older daughter, who is twelve, was brought to see me. She was complaining of the same symptoms that had plagued her parents, and suffered increased leg fatigue and foot pain after playing sports for any length of time. She also over-pronated badly, and I prescribed orthotics for her. Unlike her mother, she has worn her inserts continuously since receiving them. All her symptoms disappeared completely within two weeks of wearing them.

So, when it comes to feet, the apple often falls very close to the tree! Therefore, parents who have foot problems should watch their children carefully and have them examined immediately if the kids complain of sore legs or feet. With today's new diagnostic and treatment procedures, there is every hope that children with foot problems can be treated effectively before more serious damage occurs.

# 4

# FEMALE FEET

WHY DO WOMEN DESERVE A CHAPTER ALL TO themselves? Well, they are different, and, often, so are the foot problems they experience. This chapter focuses on conditions to which women are more prone than men and how they can avoid or treat foot problems. Designers and manufacturers of ladies' shoes are quite apt to put style before comfort and biomechanics, so women regularly don footwear that is ill suited to their feet. As a result, any biomechanical lower limb problems they may have are multiplied, and disorders they did not have originally could develop. Although a major theme of this book is that foot problems are normally caused by a biomechanical fault, I must emphasize that poorly designed, ill-fitting shoes can also induce a host of lower limb and back ailments. Because women are often disadvantaged by the inability to purchase—or choose not to purchase—proper footwear, they will develop shoe-related foot problems more frequently than men.

Many women do make an attempt to walk in comfortable shoes, at least part of the time. I must recount an incident that is related to the trend in some major North American cities for women to wear running shoes to and from work, and switch at the office to footwear more appropriate for the business world.

I was in New York three years ago with a business associate, and we noticed that a large number of women were walking along Madison Avenue in office attire and running shoes. We became curious as to how this trend began, so we decided to do a random survey of women we saw on the street. The only selection criteria were that they appeared to be between the ages of about eighteen to fifty and wore running shoes with their normal business dress.

I asked the first woman I approached if she would answer a few questions for me. She handed me a quarter and told me, quite unpolitely, to get lost. The second woman was much more friendly. She told me that the trend began in New York in 1978 when there was a public transit strike. It was uncomfortable to walk long distances in high heels, so women switched to running shoes to get to and from work and carried their pumps in a bag to change at the office. When I asked the third woman if she would answer a couple of questions she immediately said, "I'm not married, and I'm available for dinner tonight." The fourth told me that she would answer questions only from my partner. "He's cuter than you, and he's got more hair," she said. Eventually we got enough responses to confirm that the transit strike in 1978 was indeed responsible for this novel fashion statement. Since then women's athletic footwear has become a successful industry, even if the product was not always biomechanically sound.

## Vive la Différence!

Women, unlike men, have regular hormonal changes. As a result, the shape of their feet may change regularly due to fluid retention. When this happens it is especially important for them to avoid wearing tight shoes. A more monumental change occurs to a woman's body when she is pregnant, and it is of the utmost importance that she wear the proper shoes, not only for comfort but for balance as well. Have you ever seen a woman in her last trimester struggle to get around in high heels?

## Expectant Feet

As far as I know, very little has been written about how pregnancy can affect the feet. Yet many expectant women have lower limb troubles during the gestation period, and even after the baby is born. The reasons are numerous; the discomforts are not solely due to the extra burden of carrying around two additional feet.

Pregnant women must change their wardrobe as they become heavier. And yet many of them seem reluctant to change their shoes (or it never occurs to them), even when they no longer fit properly. And ill-fitting shoes are not the only problem.

The biomechanics of walking change when a woman is

pregnant. It is quite normal during the second trimester, as the expectant mother begins to gain weight, for her biomechanics to change when she is walking. Obviously, the shape of her body is being redefined. As the size of her stomach increases, her center of gravity shifts backwards, placing undue stress on the lower back. At the same time, her production of the hormones progesterone and relaxin increase dramatically.The elevated progesterone and relaxin levels relax the woman's ligaments, which become fairly flaccid and elongated, particularly in the hips to allow for the required widening of the birth canal. However, ligaments in the foot are also affected. The plantar fasciae—the long ligaments attached to the heel bone in the rearfoot and the five metatarsal bones in the forefoot—are very important in controlling over-pronation (see Diagram 6). In pregnant women these ligaments also become elongated.

An expectant mother must deal with two situations when her plantar fasciae undergo this change. Firstly, her foot will become longer. Therefore, she must switch to longer shoes, unless she is sufficiently masochistic to enjoy painfully squeezed feet. Secondly, as the plantar fasciae elongate, the feet flatten out—that is, they begin to roll more, because the ligaments have temporarily lost their ability to control pronation. So the woman can develop a wide variety of foot problems that are directly related to resulting biomechanical abnormalities. Of course, these woes should disappear once the plantar fasciae have returned to normal in the months following the delivery of the baby.

When the center of gravity of expectant mothers changes dramatically as they gain weight, they begin to develop a distinctive "pregnancy waddle"—they "toe-

*Diagram 6*
**The Plantar Fascia**

Each of the five slips descends and
embraces the flexor tendons, blending
with the tendon sheaths and the
transversed plantar metatarsal ligament

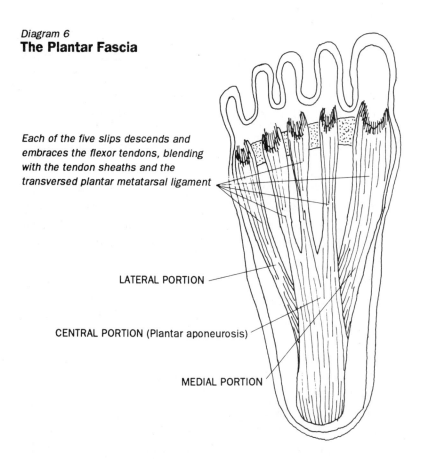

LATERAL PORTION

CENTRAL PORTION (Plantar aponeurosis)

MEDIAL PORTION

out" to maintain their balance. There is nothing unusual about this phenomenon, and their gait will return to normal once they have been delivered of their bundle of joy.

Reduced shock absorption is another reason for an expectant mother to be concerned about her feet during her pregnancy. The plantar fasciae support the longitudinal arch of the foot. When they become flaccid and longer they are no longer able to bear weight normally. Therefore, it is important for expectant mothers to wear shoes that help support the longitudinal arch. As you might have already guessed, a good pair of running shoes is the answer. If the woman continues to wear her regular footwear, she is going to have terribly tired and sore feet until long after she has delivered.

I cannot understand how a woman in her second and third trimesters can expect to walk normally in high heels. Unfortunately, I still occasionally see some expectant mothers sacrificing comfort for style. Inevitably, they pay the price. When a woman's center of gravity changes to the extent it does during pregnancy, high-heeled shoes become very uncomfortable. Imbalance and pain become the norm, because the woman's biomechanics are disastrously out of synch. The shoes cannot provide the support she so desperately requires, and her toes are being mercilessly scrunched—high-heeled shoes tend to have tight toe-boxes. So the woman becomes prone to stumbling, twisted ankles, and severe low back pain, to say nothing of her aching toes.

After the first trimester common sense is essential in the selection of footwear to avoid discomfort and biomechanical problems. Fashion shoes must be abandoned or worn only on special occasions. Even then the height of the heel should not be more than 2 inches (5 cm) and preferably of "Cuban" heel style—that is, a squarer, thicker heel.

For everyday wear nothing beats a good running shoe. It provides soft support, added shock absorption, and can prevent excessive pronation. Moreover, running shoes tend to be wider in the forefoot, and the overall width can often be increased by adjusting the lacing. This type of footwear can dramatically reduce lower limb and low back discomfort. Also, women who wear running shoes regularly can be more physically active because they may avoid many of the aches and pains often associated with the later stages of pregnancy. Legitimate medical reasons aside, there is no reason for women to be off their feet in the final trimester. Generally speaking, the fitter they are while pregnant, the easier the delivery and the quicker the recovery from childbirth.

## How Swell It Is

Many women have severe swelling (edema) in their lower extremities in the final trimester. Although there appear to be many reasons for this phenomenon, a few basic causes stand out. Firstly, the pregnant woman's kidneys are forced to function overtime and, in some cases, they become overworked and cannot filter all the fluid. As a result, excess fluid is retained in the body, and it settles in the lower limbs.

The second factor is the extra strain on the expectant mother's cardiovascular system because it must support both her and the baby. This added stress on the system adversely affects those parts of the body farthest from the heart—the lower extremities. In addition, the law of gravity forces fluids downwards, so fluid in the lower limbs cannot always be forced upwards to be filtered and eliminated. To complicate matters the uterus often inhibits the veins that are trying to return blood from the feet and legs to the heart. The lower limbs then become swollen because the cardiovascular system is unable to move fluid efficiently upwards. This situation can result in increased pressure on the veins in the legs, which contributes to the development of varicose veins, a disorder that often first appears during pregnancy.

Swelling can be controlled with proper medical care under the supervision of a family practitioner, an obstetrician-gynecologist, or other specialist. If it is allowed to continue unchecked, other problems can develop. As for the feet, swelling will obviously make otherwise perfect shoes uncomfortable. It can place tremendous pressure on, and cause extreme discomfort to, the toes by contributing to the development of soft and hard corns, hammer toes, and other conditions. It also seems to result in an increased risk of ingrown toenails: the toes become thicker and the nails dig into the expanded skin. Naturally, it is essential for women in these situations to wear proper footwear.

There are two other ways a pregnant woman can help herself. Firstly, she can wear proper-fitting support hose, which help the muscles contract when she is walking. The contracting muscles, which envelop the veins in the leg, can help the veins push the blood back up towards the heart. As a corollary of the first suggestion, a woman should walk as much as possible, unless there are medical reasons for her not to, because the exercise will help the circulation in her legs and feet.

There is one other phenomenon that I have noticed in pregnant women. Occasionally I see expectant mothers who complain of plantar warts, which are caused by the papilloma virus. I have learned over the years that these warts, which often develop in clusters, almost always disappear within a few months of giving birth, perhaps because the mother's immune system has returned to normal. My advice to these patients is to wear shoes that do not place undue stress on these warts. I will recommend aggressive treatment only if the pain becomes unbearable.

## Post-partum Foot Care

Unfortunately, foot troubles don't automatically end after a woman has given birth. It takes about six to nine months for a new mother's body to return to its normal shape. This means that her ligaments, including her plantar fasciae, are in the process of tightening. As a result, post-natal plantar fasciitis (inflammation of the plantar fasciae) is quite common for up to six months, so a woman may experience significant heel and arch pain. During this time, she should wear running shoes regularly. Not only will they provide her with increased shock absorption, they may help prevent some excessive pronation while her feet are returning to normal.

## Other Common Foot Problems

Aside from changes that occur to women's feet during pregnancy, and occasionally during the monthly cycle, their foot problems are quite similar to those of the opposite sex. Men and women of all ages can develop bunions, calluses, corns, hammer toes, neuromas, ingrown nails, and numerous other complaints. However, women often suffer more frequently from these problems because of ill-fitting shoes. The major culprit is the high-heeled shoe with the tight toe-box.

For many women, foot problems begin when they first become fashion-conscious, usually in their early teens when they are growing and definitely need proper footwear. Parents often watch helplessly while their daughters squeeze into shoes that are much too tight. Mothers are occasionally poor role models, even though they try their best to dress their children properly.

Lisa is now thirty-four and has been a patient of mine for many years. She recalls that her parents insisted she wear "orthopedic" shoes from the time she was a little girl. "They were made of the best quality leather, with good ankle and arch support," which usually meant brown, high-cut, and not particularly appealing esthetically. Unfortunately, she developed foot problems despite her parents' best intentions.

Lisa began wearing Beatle boots in her early teens, even though they were much too narrow in the toe-box for her wide feet. She was willing to endure the pain to be fashionable. Eventually her corns and calluses became unbearably sore, and she went through the entire line of over-the-counter foot care products before submitting to her mother's bathroom surgery—the razor. Her baby toes had developed hard, painful corns that did not respond to the cornucopia of over-the-counter treatments.

"As I grimaced and squirmed in pain," she recalls, "my mother, with the confidence of a surgeon, proceeded to trim off the painful corns."

Despite Mother's competence with the razor, the corns quickly reappeared, and Lisa realized by her mid-teens that there had to be another, more effective, less painful way to relieve her discomfort. She turned again to over-the-counter preparations, which she found messy and unsatisfactory. Then she came to see me.

Lisa had a wide variety of biomechanical problems that, along with her ill-fitting footwear, were causing her corns and calluses. She had begun wearing running shoes much of the time, so I prescribed a sport orthotic for her to put in her shoes. The orthotic helped support her high arches, one of the causes of her problems. She has been wearing orthotics in her shoes ever since, and her feet are basically pain-free even though she has a very active lifestyle. Although it is possible to straighten her baby toes surgically, which would remove the cause of her corns there, she has opted instead for monthly visits to my clinic to have the corns trimmed. She claims it's okay now that the "razor" is in my "very capable hands," not in her mother's.

The bunion is another problem that can be exacerbated but not caused by shoes. Contrary to popular belief, the shape of a woman's foot is not the primary cause of her bunion; nor is it the type of shoe she wears. The basic problem is one of biomechanics. Many women can wear high-heeled shoes and never develop a bunion; if shoes caused bunions, podiatrists would be able to retire early and live on the money made just from treating them. However, high-heeled shoes will definitely contribute to and worsen the discomfort of bunions, because they exaggerate pronation.

For a woman who is already an overachiever when it comes to pronation, high-heeled shoes force her toes drastically towards the inside when her forefoot is in the weight-bearing phase of her stride. This creates unbelievable stress on the big toe joint. A woman walking in a three-inch heel has her weight shifted almost directly from her heel to the ball of her foot. Her midfoot bears almost no weight at all during her stride. This is quite abnormal, and places tremendous extra pressure on the ball of her foot and, therefore, on her metatarsal bones. Excessive pressure on the big toe joint and on the head of the first metatarsal bone, a toe-box that is too small to accommodate the scrunched toes, and a woman's abnormal biomechanics together contribute to the development and discomfort of bunions.

Women are also prone to sesamoiditis, an inflammation of the area around the sesamoid bones, and stress fractures of those bones. As shown in Diagram 1, these bones sit directly under the first metatarsal bone at the big toe joint.

When women wear high-heeled shoes, the head of their first metatarsal bone tends to drop, putting tremendous stress on the underlying sesamoid bones. Computer gait analysis has revealed that there is two and a half times more weight on the sesamoids when a woman is wearing high heels than when she walks barefoot. Combine this excess weight on the sesamoids with constant walking on a hard surface, and the result can be sesamoiditis. It can be extremely painful, and is often misdiagnosed by those unfamiliar with foot problems, because of the proximity of the sesamoid bones to the big toe joint.

Fractured sesamoids are also often difficult to diagnose. A break in the bone can be detected by routine x-rays; however, about 10 to 15 per cent of people have naturally split (bipartite) sesamoid bones—a harmless, painless condition with which they were born. A stress fracture can be wrongly diagnosed because it is difficult to distinguish from a bipartite sesamoid. The presence of a fracture can be confirmed in two ways. Firstly, if a sesamoid bone is fractured, the edges of the bone will appear rough when revealed in a routine x-ray. Smooth edges would indicate that the bone is congenitally split in two and, therefore, not cracked. (It helps to look at the x-ray with a magnifying glass.) Secondly, a bone scan should be done if the medical practitioner is still unsure of the proper diagnosis. If the sesamoid is fractured a "hot spot" will appear on the scan.

Sesamoid bone problems can take time to heal properly, particularly if a fracture occurs, because of poor blood supply to that part of the foot and the constant weight-bearing stress on the bones from walking or running. Often the sesamoids do not heal; the opposing surfaces smooth off and form a "pseudo-arthrosis," which resembles a fake joint. Regardless of how the condition resolves itself, if the pain is persistent and restricts the quality of life, surgical removal of the sesamoid may be contemplated.

### The ABCs of Footwear

It is quite common for a woman to have a heel that is a narrower size than her forefoot. For example, she may have a size A heel and a size B forefoot. Until the mid-1980s designers of women's shoes usually paid little attention to the shape of a woman's foot, and the shoes they designed were often too wide in the heel, or too tight in the toe-box, or both. Very little consideration was given to comfort, since comfortable shoes seemed to be difficult to sell. Often, the prettiest shoes came in only one or two widths and were terrible fits for most of the customers. Today, I am pleased to see, greater attention is being given to making shoes that are wearable as well as attractive. However, we still have a long way to go before comfort and biomechanics replace style as the most important criteria in the design of women's footwear.

Athletic shoes for women were also less than ideal in the past. Fortunately, vast improvements have been made recently. Until the late 1980s women's running shoes were almost identical in design to men's. The same lasts were used, but the shoes were smaller. Then, three years ago, Brooks introduced Brooks for Women athletic footwear, a range of shoes combining for the first time shoe lasts designed specifically for a narrow heel and a broader forefoot. The shoes met with great success, and other athletic shoe manufacturers quickly jumped on the bandwagon. Now women can choose from a variety of well-designed athletic shoes, which will be discussed in more detail in Chapter Eight.

Women who wear high heels most of the time can develop Achilles tendinitis when they switch to athletic shoes to exercise in after years of physical inactivity. Their Achilles tendons have shrunk because they were never required to lengthen out fully when high heels were worn almost exclusively. Now the new athlete is wearing high heels to work during the day and switching to lower-heeled athletic shoes in the evening when she is exercising. Suddenly the Achilles tendon is required to stretch out sufficiently to enable her to walk, run, or jump normally in one-inch-heeled shoes. This tendon will often become inflamed, because it has become unaccustomed to stretching so far.

In addition to the Achilles tendon, the tibialis anterior and tibialis posterior muscles in the lower leg have also shrunk over the years because of the prolonged wearing of high heels. These muscles function as major anti-pronaters and also help the foot go up and down normally when it is striding. When the two muscles are required to perform tasks they can no longer handle effortlessly, they become strained, and the newly athletic woman may develop a variety of "overuse" syndromes. The most common conditions are medial and lateral shin splints, severe Achilles tendinitis, and plantar fasciitis, all of which will be discussed in detail in Chapter Seven.

### Finding the Perfect Fit

If you have a fairly normal foot, you will probably have a narrow heel and a wider forefoot. When you are shopping for a new pair of shoes, look for those that are designed with your feet in mind. They should now be easier to find in a style you like. Also, remember that any shoe with a pointed toe-box is going to scrunch your toes together. If your toes have absolutely no place to go inside the shoe, other than atop each other, you are looking for trouble. Try the following tests to determine the proper fit.

1.  Take off your right shoe, then align the sole of the left foot with the bottom of the (right) shoe. If the left foot hangs over the side of the shoe you've made the wrong choice!
2.  Trace the outline of one foot on a large piece of paper, and then cut around the tracing. Take your shoe and place it on the paper cut-out. You will probably discover that the tracing of the shoe is larger, particularly in the front.

I hope this will convince you that your shoes are too tight in the toe-box. If it doesn't, you will certainly discover the truth should you develop hard and soft corns or other forefoot problems. One of the most common of these complaints is the neuroma, which is a nerve that is pinched as it passes through the narrow confines between the toes.If the toes are scrunched together, the space through which the nerves must pass becomes even more confined. Neuromas occur most commonly between the third and fourth toes, and can be quite painful, particularly when a woman is wearing high-heeled shoes. It would seem logical to me that a woman ought to sacrifice a bit of fashion for the sake of comfort. Unfortunately, it often takes an excruciatingly painful neuroma episode for that logic to hit home.

Women who suffer from PMS (premenstrual syndrome) should buy at least one larger pair of fashion shoes to wear when their feet swell because they are retaining water. Support hose may also help during PMS; they are no longer as unattractive as they once were. Running shoes are ideal at this time, because the toe-box is larger and the width can be increased by loosening the laces.

### On Her Toes

Most women take pride in well-groomed feet, particularly their toes. Therefore, they often treat themselves to a pedicure every now and then, especially if they regularly wear open-toed shoes.

Pedicures have been around for centuries, as have painted toenails, which can make a fashion statement in their own right. However, nail polish ought to be avoided when a woman develops one or more fungal nails. Fungus flourishes best in the dark, particularly when not exposed to sunlight. If a woman's toenail has been attacked by a fungal infection, and if she then paints that nail with polish, she is effectively blocking out light that may slow down or possibly impede growth of the fungus. If you are a woman who constantly wears high-heeled shoes, particularly ones that are very tiny in the toe-box, you may be in for some nasty surprises. If you suddenly decide to take up a physical activity and begin wearing athletic shoes after having worn primarily heels for years, you may also develop foot problems. And if you refuse to wear proper shoes when you are pregnant, you may open yourself up to a cornucopia of aches and pains from the lower back down to your toes. So a word to the wise: Be sensible about your footwear and you will save yourself a lot of misery.

# 5

# VARICOSE VEINS

THE SCOPE OF PODIATRY DOES NOT NORMALLY extend to varicose veins. But scopes have broadened and lengthened over the years, particularly in the medical profession. The causes of and treatment for varicose veins are numerous, and the two common procedures usually used to eliminate them are controversial. I have consulted with medical colleagues who are well versed in this condition, and I intend to share with you the fruits of my labor. By the end of this chapter you should have a solid layperson's knowledge of varicose veins—perhaps more than you ever wanted to know—which ought to allay all the myths and fears associated with the disorder.

## Arteries and Veins
Contrary to popular opinion, varicose veins are not an

indication of poor cardiovascular circulation. Cardiovascular disorders generally involve the malfunction of the arteries, which carry fresh blood from the heart to all parts of the body. The oxygen that is supplied by the lungs, and which is responsible for keeping our organs and tissues alive, is distributed throughout the body by the blood, propelled by the heart through the arteries and their tributaries, the arterioles. When arteries narrow or become clogged, or when the heart is somehow damaged and cannot pump efficiently, a sufficient supply of fresh blood cannot be delivered to the body, and particularly to the outer extremities, such as the feet.

Veins and their tributaries, the venuoles, pick up de-oxygenated blood from capillaries, which pass blood from the arterial system to the venous system, and return it to the heart. Because the heart is pumping fresh blood out to the body, a different mechanism is required to return "spent" blood to it for re-oxygenation. So, veins are provided with valves that open and close with each heartbeat. Unlike the arteries, the veins have no muscle fibers in their linings to help propel the blood towards its destination. Therefore, the role of these venous valves is vital.

The two major superficial veins that originate in the foot and travel up the leg are the long saphenous (internal) vein and the short saphenous (external) vein. The former runs from the forefoot and up the big toe side of the foot on the inside of the leg; the latter begins on the outside part of the forefoot and runs up the back of the leg. There are also two deeper veins, the posterior and anterior tibial veins, and numerous auxiliary veins that feed into the major vessels. These smaller veins become important when the valves of the major ones become defective.

The long and short saphenous veins are the ones most often affected by valve dysfunction, which can lead to the condition we call varicose veins. The valves malfunction for many reasons, not the least of which is pregnancy. (This is why the incidence of varicose veins is higher in women than in men. Once the damage has been done, the valves cannot naturally repair themselves.) Whatever the cause, an over-stressed valve becomes unable to handle the volume of blood that is trying to return to the heart. Blood then backs up in the vein, because it cannot get through the valve and up to the heart. In the case of pregnancy, the pressure of the fetus on the pelvis can directly impair valve function of the femoral vein and, indirectly, the long saphenous vein. As the pressure of the fetus on the pelvis increases, the thin-walled veins can develop an "outpouch," similar to an air pocket or bubble you would find in a defective tire. This outpouching can create a discoloration that is most apparent when the affected vein is close to the skin.

Blood that has lost its oxygen supply has a bluish tinge. Therefore, varicose veins are blue because they contain spent blood trying to return to the heart. The blood has backed up because the valves in the veins are unable to function normally, and it has settled in the outpouches while it searches for another vein with normal valves to return it to the heart. Once a varicose vein condition has developed it will not simply repair itself; outpouches do not heal naturally with time.

## Non-surgical Treatment of Varicose Veins
Varicose veins are not life-threatening; nature

automatically forces the blood to seek alternative vessels that will take it back to the heart. However, the condition can become uncomfortable and esthetically unappealing. These smaller alternative veins, which are closer to the skin, were not designed to carry such a large volume of blood, so they too can develop outpouches. This may be quite painful and can create ugly discoloration. If the discomfort becomes unbearable, surgery may be the only answer. Otherwise, the person can either learn to live with the "blues" or take steps to control the damage.

An ounce of prevention is worth pounds of cure. Women could avoid pregnancy, although this is a rather drastic step to take. Obesity is a factor that could be avoided. Heavier people automatically place a greater strain on their cardiovascular systems, which may eventually affect the ability of the valves in the veins to function normally. Workers who must stand for long periods may also place undue stress on the veins, as their muscles eventually tighten from fatigue. Veins pass through the same areas as these muscles and can be adversely affected by the cramping. So work habits ought to be changed to allow workers either to walk or sit for a time during the day. Some people have been genetically cursed with poor valve function and are naturally prone to varicose veins. They can control their fate to a certain extent by avoiding obesity, work that requires them to stand for a long time in one spot, and, in the extreme, pregnancy. There is also one other remedial step they can take.

## The First Line of Defence
The least expensive and invasive treatment by far for varicose veins is wearing support hose. It was originally

thought that support hose wrap the lower legs like a tensor bandage and reduce outpouching because the valves in the veins do not have to strain so much to force the blood back towards the heart. However, the weakness—like a hernia—remains, although it is kept somewhat under control. The concept has not really changed: providing they are not too tight, the support hose help the veins function better, because they compress the veins and encourage flow back to the heart, and prevent swelling, which is associated with leg fatigue. If the support hose are too tight, they will cramp the muscles and impede proper circulation.

### Doc the Stripper

If a person with varicose veins decides on an invasive solution to his or her problem because of discomfort or for cosmetic reasons, there are two major options to consider. The oldest and most common of these is vein stripping. Peripheral-vascular surgeons (those who operate on blood vessels not directly connected to the heart) strip malfunctioning veins, usually the long saphenous and its auxiliaries, which are the ones most likely to become varicose.

The thought of vein stripping may not be all that appealing to you once you learn how it's done. Yet it can be effective, and the procedure is simple and quick, although the recovery period may be uncomfortable and lengthy.

As shown in Diagram 7, a cut is made in the groin area to where the long saphenous vein begins. The junction of the long saphenous vein with the femoral vein is identified, and the branches of the long saphenous vein are tied off

Diagram 7
## The Long and Short Saphenous Veins and Their Branches

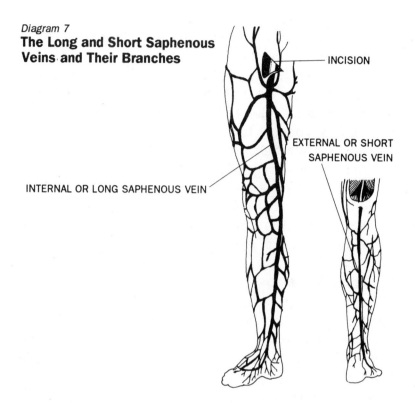

INCISION

EXTERNAL OR SHORT SAPHENOUS VEIN

INTERNAL OR LONG SAPHENOUS VEIN

to help avoid recurrence. A second incision is made in the ankle, and the long saphenous vein is identified. A plastic wire is then inserted into the vein at the ankle and passed up towards the groin. If passage is difficult, at least one additional incision is made along the course of the vein to aid the upward movement of the wire. Once the wire reaches the groin a screw-on "acorn" is attached to it at the lower end of the vein—at the ankle—thereby sealing off the vein at the ankle. The surgeon grabs the top of the wire at the head of the long saphenous vein and quickly pulls it and the "acorn" up and out. The rapid action effectively removes the vein from the body without ripping away an excess amount of tissue surrounding the vein.

The body quickly reacts to replace the function of the stripped long saphenous vein. The blood seeks out other veins and venuoles through which it can pass up towards the heart. It will take a while for these alternative vessels to completely take up the slack, but eventually blood flow from the feet and legs to the heart should return to normal as the veins naturally enlarge to handle the task.

Varicose veins can return after vein stripping if valve problems develop in the vessels that have accepted the greater work load. The person should take preventive steps, as discussed above, to lessen the risks of further outpouching. In fact, it might occasionally be wiser to live with the original condition; the veins with the damaged valves may still be performing sufficiently to relieve the pressure on other veins in the area. If the alternative veins are unable to pick up the slack created by the removal of the stripped veins, the person may develop considerable lower leg swelling (edema).

Scarring is the second side effect of varicose vein surgery. Depending on the number of veins stripped and the technique of the surgeon, the patient will be left with at least two scars, each nearly an inch (2 cm) long. So, if varicose vein sufferers do not experience a lot of pain or swelling of the lower extremities, they will have to decide if surgery for cosmetic reasons is practical. They may be eliminating one color (blue) for another (angry red).

### Injections: Often in Vain?

There has been much controversy in the past few years about the benefits of injecting a varicose vein to destroy it rather than removing it surgically.

A varicose vein is given a series of injections with a sclerosing agent, which destroys the vein without the need for more invasive, scarring surgery. Sclerosis is a hardening of tissue and is often associated with diseases such as multiple sclerosis and atherosclerosis. If a vein can no longer function adequately and has become varicose, intentionally sclerosing it by causing it to become inflamed and scarred can be an alternative to surgery.

Unfortunately, injection treatment does not always solve the underlying problems associated with varicose veins, nor can it be used on the major veins in the lower extremities, because of the difficulty in non-invasively isolating the exact areas to be injected and because of their higher blood flow. It seems to be most useful for small, superficial (spider) veins that develop valve problems and outpouches. The sclerosing agent can be injected into these small localized areas, and the tiny veins collapse permanently. There is no scarring or discoloration after the procedure—only temporary bruising—so the results are more esthetically pleasing than surgery. However, many medical experts believe that the injections are merely a short-term solution, because the problem may lie with a larger, deeper vein, and other, smaller veins in the area will eventually become varicose as well.

Determining if you might be a suitable candidate for the injection of a sclerosing agent will depend to a large extent on whether the valves in the larger veins in your legs are functioning normally. That decision can be made with the help of diagnostic tests. If the valves aren't functioning normally, and if you require treatment for your condition, a surgical solution may be your only choice. On the other hand, if only a few small, superficial veins are involved you may find your answer lies in the needle. Keep in mind that there is no guarantee that your varicose vein problems are over after you have been injected.

There are no miracle, completely non-invasive cures for varicose veins. An invasive cure may be less comforting and effective than a commonsense approach to living with them. Whatever your decision, I suggest that you obtain more than one expert opinion of your particular situation before you make up your mind.

# 6

# GERIATRIC FEET

DEMOGRAPHICS AND DEMANDS ON THE HEALTH care systems in North America are changing. Our population is slowly aging, and geriatric foot care will become increasingly important as we hurtle towards the next century. This chapter is devoted to foot problems often faced by our senior citizens and to a discussion of a logical exercise regimen for them. With the proper training program they ought to be able to stay in shape, and feel good at the same time.

## The Geriathlete
Although not everyone of retirement age is able to undertake

a fitness regimen, there is no reason for the average senior to abstain from physical activity, which need not involve running a marathon or playing squash non-stop for two hours. However, there are a few hurdles to jump, and just as many hangups to overcome.

When it comes to physical activity, seniors fall into several categories. The two I propose to discuss are those who have never seriously exercised, and those who have always been physically active but are afraid to slow down because they believe it is an admission of aging.

The first category includes previously inactive seniors who may want to begin an exercise program but are reluctant to start. These people hesitate for various reasons. Many are too embarrassed to seek help. They believe they are too old, or too out of shape; they feel insecure watching their juniors work out, and guilty for having led a sedentary life in their younger days. Others are frightened. They fear that they might drop dead on the spot from a heart attack when they begin exercising, or that they will make a spectacle of themselves. They think athletes will laugh at them; they are afraid of wearing the wrong clothing or footwear, which could also be an embarrassment. Finally, there are those who just don't know where or how to begin. Should they join a fitness studio or the local Y? What type of exercises should they be doing? Who can best instruct them?

On the flip side of this coin are the geriatrics who believe they can just begin exercising without first ascertaining their physical condition and determining what exercise program is best for them. These are the people who may suffer a heart attack the first time they take to the track or the gym, because their cardiovascular systems cannot handle the sudden surge of extra stress. Many of them have never exercised a day in their lives or have not worked out in years. Some have been heavy smokers or drinkers, and are overweight with high blood pressure. Others may be in decent health but are totally unprepared for the rigors of a strenuous new exercise regimen.

The second category includes those who have been physically active all their lives. Such people may have run an average of sixty miles a week and a couple of marathons a year. They may have also indulged a few hours a week in other strenuous activities, for example by playing squash or tennis, or by working out in a gym. Now they find themselves unable to maintain such a vigorous schedule, no matter how hard they push themselves. They are terribly afraid to admit they are growing older, but their bodies have indeed aged and are no longer able to cope with the physical punishment. Bones and joints have naturally become worn; muscles and other soft tissues require more time to recuperate from the stress of hard exercise. They must slow down, but fear doing so and are ill informed about fitness programs suitable for older people.

Seniors in both categories need some basic commonsense rules. For those of you who have never exercised, the most important step is learning how to get started. I strongly believe that any beginner over thirty-five should first have a physical examination, including a proper stress test, which, 80 per cent of the time, will indicate any heart problems that might be activated or exacerbated by strenuous physical activity.

If the examination indicates that you are in good shape, your doctor will give you the green light to begin a sensible program of physical activity. The knowledge that you appear to be healthy should allay your fears about starting an exercise program even though you may have reached retirement age. Even if you are not 100 per cent convinced, remember that a sedentary lifestyle hardly guarantees a long life. You are much better off getting out to smell the roses rather than sitting in your favorite armchair and watching them wilt in the vase.

Once you have been given the green light to proceed, the next step is to choose the type of exercise that is right for you. Some people hate running; others have no use for the water, or cannot swim. There are those who enjoy privacy and those who like group activities. Whichever form of exercise you choose, the important thing to remember is to practise moderation. A few geriathletes can run marathons or cross-country ski 50 miles a day, but they are the exception rather than the norm.

My first choice as an activity for seniors is walking. Walking has been called the perfect exercise. It is something most people do daily; in fact, if you are sixty-five you have been walking for at least sixty-three years, so you know you are not venturing into some new physical endeavor that might be physically harmful. The speed can be adjusted to suit your needs; there is less wear and tear on the bones and joints than in other forms of exercise (with the exception of swimming); it is an excellent form of cardiovascular activity; it can be done anywhere, anytime, either alone or with others; there are no schedules to follow or expensive clubs to join; the only equipment required is appropriate clothing and good walking or running shoes; and there are no fancy techniques to learn. It does not matter whether you walk indoors or outside. If the weather is particularly inclement, you can join other seniors who are often found striding purposefully through the long corridors of apartment buildings and shopping malls.

Some of you may want to run or jog, which is fine as long as you are physically able to do so. (The difference between running and jogging is generally considered to be eight minutes. If you can do a mile in eight minutes or less—or 1 km in five minutes or less—you are running; otherwise you are deemed to be jogging.) Since some people can walk a mile comfortably in a little over ten minutes, walking may actually be better than jogging, because it places less stress on the body. Younger people usually start by jogging and gradually build up to running. However, if you are a senior citizen and have never run before, I would suggest that you stick to walking. You won't suffer the aches and pains of a new jogger, which means that you won't be too discouraged by the discomfort to continue with the program.

As for the geriathlete who cannot accept the facts of aging, I have some sound advice. Listen to what your body is telling you before the only thing you hear is pain and suffering. You don't have to call it quits altogether, but unless you are an exceptional individual, you should not be in training for a triathlon. I know of one person who took at least two brisk twenty-minute walks a day until well into his late nineties. He never undertook any other physical activity and was as fit when a nonagenarian as he had been when he reached retirement age.

One of my favorite patients is a seventy-one-year-old man who has managed to lead a moderately active life despite a multitude of foot and leg problems. He is a wonderful example of a senior who has not allowed the aging process and non-life-threatening disorders to force him to abandon all types of physical activity. He is also well aware of the limitations of his body, and, with proper medical supervision, follows a sensible daily routine. He walks as much as he can.

John first came to my office a few months ago with a litany of ailments—calluses, hammer toes, a bunion and a bunionette (on a baby toe), osteoarthritis, rheumatoid arthritis (now in remission), varicose veins, and some circulatory dysfunction in his feet. His condition has been exacerbated over the years by a combination of neglect, poliomyelitis, naval war service, which left him with unmended broken toes, a moderate case of immersion foot (exposure to cold, but less severe than frostbite), and the constant wearing of ill-fitting shoes.

Before he was sent to me, John had run the gamut of medical care—from medical doctors to physiotherapists—with varying results and, at times, was in such excruciating pain in his lower extremities that he suffered, he says, episodes of "rapidly deteriorating physical and mental condition." He has become a regular patient. As he describes his visits to either me or my chiropodist, they consist of "artistic carving, orthotic device adjustments, pedicures, and an exchange of jokes and baseball news." John is much happier now because he has regained a more active lifestyle, thanks to orthotics and regular appointments to trim his calluses and corns to ensure that he does not develop new biomechanical problems.

According to John, the "medical advice and continued supervision of my foot program, and more recently the addition of orthotics, has not healed or cured the problems.

But it has effected considerable and continuing relief from pain and discomfort, a major improvement in mobility and, to date, prevented any damage to upper joints and back as a result of improved balance."

John is careful not to attempt the physical feats of a younger man. A seventy-year-old body cannot withstand physical punishment so well as a younger body. Muscles take longer to rebound from strenuous usage; joints are often no longer able to tolerate the stress of continuous exercising. In some people, particularly women, bones become brittle and may break if overstressed. These are undeniable facts of nature. Therefore, common sense dictates that when we get older we adopt a physical fitness program more suited to our bodies' limitations.

Those who have been physically active all their lives should continue with the same basic exercise regimen they have enjoyed for years. They may shorten their routines, particularly if they begin to suffer nagging aches and pains. Runners who start experiencing discomforts in their lower extremities should have the biomechanics of their legs and feet checked by an expert to avoid serious low back, hip, knee, and foot problems. Some foot faults do not show up until a person has reached middle age, and are often overlooked as a cause of pain in other parts of the body.

Proper footwear is essential for all geriathletes, and many of them may require shoe inserts, such as orthotics, to prevent foot abnormalities from becoming serious problems. As I have previously mentioned, good walking or running shoes are required. I recommend sticking to the leading manufacturers, including Nike, Brooks, Saucony, New Balance, and Reebok.

### Sock It to Me!

As people age their skin becomes more sensitive. Therefore they are more prone to irritations, inflammations, and blistered feet. Part of the problem is the natural aging process of the skin. Another factor is that seniors usually have reduced circulation in their lower extremities, which means that they take longer to recover from a foot problem or injury because their blood is not delivering healing nutrients to the affected area quickly enough or in sufficient amounts, as it did at a younger age. (I shall have more to say about circulatory problems in Chapter Nine.)

One simple way to prevent or reduce these problems is to wear the proper socks, particularly when you are exercising. Natural fibers such as wool and cotton absorb moisture much better than synthetic fabrics, such as nylon. When you walk or otherwise exercise, your feet perspire. If you aren't wearing two- or three-layer cotton or wool socks, that sweat will not be absorbed and your feet will become quite moist. This is an ideal way for them to become irritated. Moreover, they can become breeding grounds for the growth of fungal infections. It doesn't matter if you wear athletic socks, tube socks, or fancy knee-length argyles, just so long as they fit properly and absorb moisture effectively.

### Listen Up

Now that you are properly attired, let's get back to your exercise regimen. First a reminder that if you refuse to listen to what your body is telling you, and continue to attempt an exercise program that is unsuitable for an older person, you could be in for big trouble. As you have already heard, the foot bones are indirectly connected to the back bones. If you keep trying to run ten miles a day on legs and feet that can no longer tolerate the constant pounding, the overstress can be felt from your toes up to your spine. All the bones and joints in between are also being jarred; muscles and other soft tissues are being stressed and may become inflamed. And, if you try to exercise through the pain, the discomfort will only get worse. Eventually you will have to postpone your athletic endeavors and seek medical attention. Sometimes the recovery period is lengthy, and you may become disillusioned. If that happens you may give up all forms of activity altogether, much to the detriment of your long-term physical and emotional well-being.

Before I discuss how to avoid injuries, I want to stress the marvelous sense of relaxation and well-being a person can experience after even a mild form of exercise. This state of emotional wellness has been fully documented in popular and professional literature, and I urge all seniors who are physically able to learn  for themselves the positive qualities of exercise. I am also constantly amazed by the number of older patients who tell me that their aches and pain seem to ease or vanish completely after they have begun a sensible exercise regimen. Not only are they physically better, they also experience substantial drops in anxiety levels. They speak of a vastly improved quality of life they had not enjoyed in years. I recently heard of one man who had suffered for years from terrible hip pain. He began an exercise program a few months ago, which was designed to develop muscle tone and strength without straining any of the weight-bearing joints of the body. He now claims to be almost totally free of his hip pain, without the use of any drugs.

Over the years I have had numerous conversations with Dr. Robbie Wolfe, a teaching cardiologist at the University of Toronto. He strongly believes that almost all people with internal diseases would benefit from a more active daily lifestyle. He points, as examples, to diabetics and people with cardiovascular diseases. It was thought for years that diabetics and persons with vascular disease (which includes poor blood flow to the feet, and also affects diabetics) should lead sedentary lives. The same applied to heart disease patients, who often literally wasted away after suffering some form of cardiac incident. This theory has now been completely disproved, and many heart attack victims have recovered to run in marathons. In fact, in 1990 a heart transplant recipient completed the Boston Marathon—a race more than twenty-six miles long! So there is hope for everyone, even those who have suffered major cardiovascular incidents. And many rehabilitation programs begin with walking. This is why it is so important that the first walking experience be comfortable and pleasant. If your lower extremities hurt during or after you begin your regimen, you may give up exercising altogether. What a shame that would be.

Dr. Wolfe agrees that the first activity a heart patient should undertake is a walking program. This program, which can eventually lead to jogging or running, should be devised by qualified personnel and cardiovascular rehabilitation centers, which can be found in almost all urban communities. Dr. Nathan Pritikin, who was one of the world's leading nutritional experts before he died a few years ago, demanded that his patients undertake an exercise program along with his diet regimen to achieve maximum benefit from the program.

Now that you are firmly convinced you will become a geriathlete, let's discuss how you can avoid the pitfalls of incorrect exercising. If you have no major aches and pains to begin with, and you want to stay that way, you must remember one basic truth: The older you get, the more slowly your body recovers from athletic stress. Your muscles, for example, will take longer to return to normal after exercise than when you were younger. However, any post-exercise discomfort can be significantly reduced or eliminated by taking the proper precautions. The first step is to warm up and stretch properly before walking, running, or doing any other form of exercise.

Many excellent books can teach you how to warm up and stretch correctly. If you are receiving special medical attention, a qualified athletic therapist will devise a program for you. One of the problems addressed by such programs is the buildup in the muscles of lactic acid, which appears to be the primary cause of post-exercise aches and pains. The abundance of lactic acid in the muscles is much more prevalent after anaerobic exercise (the type that does not specifically promote the increase of heart/lung function) than aerobic exercise (which is designed to increase cardiopulmonary function). It is also much more common in seniors than in younger people, and takes longer—24 to 48 hours—to dissipate, particularly in those people who have not exercised regularly in years. There is no doubt, however, that a proper warm-up, stretch, walking/running, stretch, and cool-down will greatly alleviate the lactic acid problem, regardless of the athlete's age. Therefore, it is vital for new geriathletes to learn how to prepare their bodies properly for their walking program.

### Osteoarthritis

A problem that commonly occurs along with the aging process is osteoarthritis. It is important for the geriathlete to understand just what osteoarthritis is and how exercise programs can help reduce, rather than increase, the discomfort.

Despite recent studies that may indicate a disease component, I maintain that osteoarthritis is not a disease. It is a wear-and-tear process that affects the joints of the body, and is exacerbated by abnormal biomechanics. As an analogy, think of the tires on your automobile. If the wheels are out of alignment, the surfaces of the tires will ride unevenly on the road, and the tread will wear out faster wherever each tire is absorbing an abnormal amount of shock. In normal conditions, the tires will wear evenly and over a much longer time than if the wheels are unbalanced. Similarly, if you are walking "unbalanced," you are placing undue stress on certain joints in your lower extremities. If you are striding normally—with or without the aid of orthotic devices—your joints should remain normal, although some natural wear and tear will probably occur as you get older.

When your joints are abnormally stressed, the cartilage that prevents bone from rubbing against bone becomes frayed or worn out. At the same time the joint capsule loses the synovial fluid that lubricates the joint. As a result an inflammation occurs, and eventually bone may begin rubbing against bone, thereby causing constant, often excruciating pain.

There is good news and bad news when it comes to osteoarthritis. First the bad. If you wait too long to deal with the problem, you may require surgery or medication to alleviate the discomfort. Also, you may settle into a sedentary lifestyle that you will most likely find far from rewarding.

The good news is that prompt, correct treatment can prevent osteoarthritis from worsening, and may even reverse the progress of the condition. Medical experts are now convinced that proper, moderate exercise can help in the regeneration of cartilage and synovial fluid in a joint. This is what apparently happened to the man with the bad hips, who benefited greatly from his exercise regiment. So rather than retiring for life from physical activity because of osteoarthritis, a person can now take simple, non-invasive, non-medicated steps to defeat it. The key words here are proper and moderate. (There is also evidence that exercise may slow or actually prevent the onset of osteoporosis, a condition most prevalent in post-menopausal women and one that results in extremely brittle bones.)

One of the most common sites of osteoarthritis in seniors is the medial compartment of the knee (see Diagram 8). If a person is slightly bowlegged he will place excess weight on the inside (medial) part of the knee. As the years go by the increased stress will wear down the cartilage at that part of the knee joint. Moreover, unless the abnormality is corrected, his bowleggedness will increase. Also, if he becomes heavier he will place even greater stress on the medial compartment of the knee, thereby exacerbating further his osteoarthritic condition. This is because bone always conforms to stress—that is, it will grow or move in a certain direction to alleviate a dysfunction. Eventually, the pain will become so debilitating that surgery may be required.In fact, until recently it was

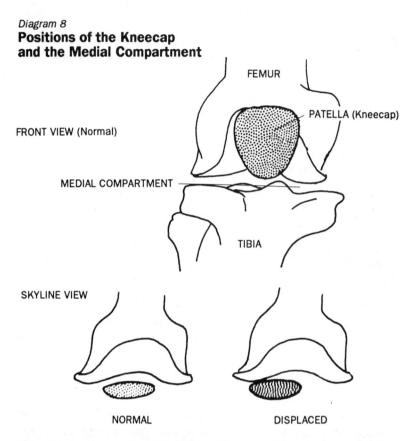

*Diagram 8*
**Positions of the Kneecap
and the Medial Compartment**

FEMUR

PATELLA (Kneecap)

FRONT VIEW (Normal)

MEDIAL COMPARTMENT

TIBIA

SKYLINE VIEW

NORMAL

DISPLACED

the primary course of action. The operation was called a high tibial osteotomy, which involves cutting a wedge-shaped piece of bone out of the tibia just below the knee. When the bone heals it will be straight. As a result the person will no longer walk bowlegged, and the excess pressure on the medial compartment of the knee will be relieved.

As you can imagine, a high tibial osteotomy is not minor surgery, and the recovery time will be measured in weeks and months rather than in days. This is particularly true for seniors, since they do not naturally heal as quickly as younger people. So, wouldn't it be wonderful if such surgery could be avoided!

There is hope for people with medial compartment osteoarthritis: a treatment program that includes orthotics, specially designed exercise programs, and weight loss. It is certainly worth a try, considering the alternatives—surgery or debilitating pain. The success rate of this non-invasive approach will depend on the extent of the damage already done to the knee joint. Therefore, the sooner this treatment program is begun the better the chance of success.

Back to exercise regimens. If you suffer from severe knee or hip osteoarthritis, you may initially find walking too difficult. There are other forms of movement that will allow you to exercise without having to bear any weight on the affected joints. Swimming is the most notable example, though there are others for those who aren't comfortable in the water. However, if you are able to walk without significant discomfort, and your condition has been confirmed by a medical professional to be osteoarthritis, you should consider a walking program. You may be amazed by the positive results.

To minimize joint or soft tissue pain, you must start your walking program sensibly. By that I mean slowly. Let us assume that you are wearing the correct footwear. Now, begin your walk at a leisurely pace to warm up. After a few minutes, take time out to stretch your muscles. A number of excellent exercise books can show you the proper stretching routines. Then walk a bit more briskly for a few minutes. (Don't overdo it! If you feel tired or achy, stop!) After you have finished your walk—which should ideally be near your starting point—stretch out the muscles again while they are still warm. Then you can cool down by walking leisurely for a couple of minutes. Initially, you ought to walk only on alternate days so that you allow your muscles and joints to recuperate, because they are not yet accustomed to any form of exercise.

Before turning to other foot problems often faced by seniors,I want to remind you of what I said at the beginning of this chapter. Every new geriathlete must have a complete physical examination before undertaking an exercise program. And every geriathlete must have the proper footwear, and follow a specific regimen suited to his or her needs.Remember that an educated consumer is most often a happy one. If you are unsure about what type of shoes to wear or exercise program to undertake, don't be afraid to seek expert advice. Above all, don't waste your golden years sitting on your hands. Get up onto your feet and enjoy life!

## On the Nail

Often as you get older you have trouble bending over to examine and care for your feet. So, until they begin to bother you, you tend not to fuss with them. Unfortunately, if you do not pay attention to your feet, they may cause you considerable pain.

One of the most common problems with the geriatric foot is the fungal nail. More than half of my geriatric patients have at least one fungal nail, because seniors are naturally more susceptible to foot inflammations and infections. They also often fail to realize that they have traumatized a toe, and that a bit of blood may have pierced the skin under the nail. So they should watch for the appearance of a dark spot (dried blood) under their nails. Fungi thrive in dark, moist, warm environments. They are nourished by the bit of blood under the nail, and revel in the warmth and darkness of a foot covered by a shoe. If the owner of the toe is not wearing the proper socks, and perspiration stays on the foot rather than soaking into the stocking, so much the better for the fungi.

A fungal nail is distinguished by its yellowish discoloration; as well, it will begin to detach itself from the nail bed. The symptoms can take up to three to six months to appear, by which time the infection will have grabbed a solid toe-hold and may be difficult to eliminate. Fortunately, the condition is not often painful, although the nail may not be pretty to look at. The fungus can often be kept under control with the help of anti-fungal creams; however, it may have affected the nail-growing cells, which means that the infection could return. If, as occasionally happens, the condition becomes painful and untreatable, the nail can be removed and the nail-growing cells destroyed without too much discomfort to the patient. He or she will then be left with a nail-less but painless toe.

Another nail problem that can affect the geriatric toe is onychogryphosis, which is an all-encompassing medical term for thick, distorted nails. These nails have become thicker and harder to cut for a variety of reasons, the most common being constant trauma to the toes from years of wear and tear and the wearing of ill-fitting shoes (particularly high heels with tiny toe-boxes). Abnormalities develop if damage has been done to the nail bed and nail-growing cells of the toe. If the toe doesn't hurt, leave it alone. Routine nail care by a podiatrist, including grinding the nail to make it thinner, may help prevent a worsening of the condition. Should the area become painful, the nail may have to be removed and the nail bed destroyed. The treatment sounds worse than it really is; the procedure is similar to the modern technique for painlessly removing ingrown toenails, and the toe should heal fairly quickly, with no return of the discomfort.

### Drying Out
We all know that as we age our skin gets drier. The dry skin on our feet, particularly the heels, can crack and become quite uncomfortable; it also becomes more susceptible to inflammations and infections. The solution to this problem lies in moisturizing creams. There is no need to spend a fortune—an inexpensive one will do the trick quite nicely. The only potential problem would be an allergy to the product you are using, so you might want to read labels carefully before you buy anything.

### When Fat Is Fit
One of the nasty truths of aging is that nature tends to reverse what was normal when we were in our prime. Hair no longer grows where it should and grows where it shouldn't; what should be hard becomes soft and vice versa; fat disappears from where it belongs and appears where we don't want it. This last situation is what concerns us here.

The ball of the foot is where the heads of the metatarsal bones are joined to the base of the toe bones. The medical term for the area is the transverse metatarsal arch. If you were to examine the ball of an infant's foot you would find a big wad of fat there to protect the developing bones from injury. As the child begins to walk that fat pad diminishes sufficiently to allow for balance. Slowly, as we progress from childhood to old age, that fat pad thins out. Sometimes it thins out more quickly if a person is suffering from certain diseases, such as rheumatoid arthritis or diabetes. A thinning fat pad has become more prevalent over the years because we are living longer, and often reaches the point where it disappears.When this happens people complain that the bones in their feet seem to be on the verge of bursting through their skin. Fortunately, the underlying skin is sufficiently dense to prevent such an unpleasant occurrence. However, every step these people take can be excruciatingly painful, because the bones on the balls of the feet are now directly exposed to pressure each time they bear weight—which is with every stride.There is nothing to cushion the bones from this constant pounding, and the area becomes inflamed.The pain is enhanced because the nerve endings on the bottom of the feet are close to the surface of the skin.

There are various ways of dealing with disappearing fat pads. One approach is to inject the area with medical-grade collagen, which acts as a replacement for the fat pad. However, the collagen usually breaks down after six to twelve months, so it must be reinjected regularly. If you are not squeamish about needles, you might consider collagen as an alternative to suffering for the rest of your life.

The most logical approach is to relieve the area of excessive weight-bearing stress.Often, shoe inserts—such as Spenco or Sorbathane insoles—will provide some relief and eliminate the need for more aggressive action, such as custom-made orthotics. Best of all is a running shoe that provides a spongy underpad, which should absorb sufficient shock to enable the person to walk pain-free. I have found that the two types of shoe that best replace a lost fat pad are the Nike Air and the Brooks HydroFlow (filled with water). (I will discuss these shoes in detail in Chapter Eight.)

One of my patients, an active eighty-two-year-old man, came to me two years ago with all the symptoms I mentioned above. He had almost no fat pad left on either foot, and could not walk more than a few yards before experiencing excruciating pain where the bones were exposed. I ordered a pair of orthotics for him and advised him to buy a pair of Spenco insoles for his shoes while he was waiting for the orthotics. He obtained appreciable relief with the Spenco inserts he purchased, and now switches back and forth between them and the orthotics, depending on the shoes he is wearing. The bottoms of his feet rarely hurt him any more.

I hope that all seniors who read this chapter, and who are sufficiently healthy to undertake a moderate exercise program, will realize that there is no need for them to become sedentary after they have reached retirement age. Pay closer attention to your feet so that you can avoid or at least alleviate some of the conditions I have described. If you are unable to care for your feet yourself, have them examined and cared for periodically. Treat yourself to a pedicure once in a while—and that goes for men as well! If you take good care of your feet, they will help keep you active and happy for a long time.

# 7

# OVERUSED AND ABUSED FROM BACK TO FOOT

WHEN I FIRST WROTE ABOUT OVERUSE SYNDROMES I concentrated primarily on the difficulties encountered by athletes. In this chapter I will update information I have previously discussed. I wish to focus on problems that are much more prevalent today and are not specifically related to athletic activities. I also look at many of the recent fashionable forms of exercise and their relationships with lower limb disorders. And, of course, I will continually emphasize the connection between the feet and other parts of the body, up to the lower back.

As a podiatrist, I focus on motion when I see a patient with an apparent biomechanical problem. Biomechanics is very much a science. I must observe and evaluate the information I receive from watching the patient walk or run, and interpret the findings of computer gait analysis. If, for example, a patient has a knee problem, I have to determine from a mechanical point of view if there is a cause-and-effect relationship between the foot and the knee. An orthopedic specialist, on the other hand, will analyze findings from a medical examination of the patient, and the symptoms, to determine the cause of the complaint. So I am searching for a mechanical problem; the orthopod is looking more for an organic disorder. The true art of biomechanics is the knowledge of the correlation between organic and mechanical dysfunction, which is why I work closely with orthopedic experts at the Sports Medicine Clinic of the Mount Sinai Hospital and at the Canadian Back Institute.

The inability to diagnose correctly an overuse or other foot-related problem occurs when the sciences of medicine and biomechanics fail to interact to find the cause of the trouble. Therefore, it is essential that the person with an apparent overuse injury understand the relationships between the various parts of the anatomy. A simple way of determining whether your discomfort is caused by an organic or a biomechanical problem is to buy a pair of good running shoes. If after walking or running in them your condition improves significantly, you can conclude fairly safely that your troubles are biomechanical. On the other hand, if new shoes make absolutely no difference, you may have an organic problem, and you should seek prompt medical attention.

## Run-down Runners

One of the catalysts in the rapid advances in the analysis and treatment of foot and leg disorders was the running craze that exploded in the 1970s. Athletic and physical therapists began seeing large numbers of runners and joggers with a host of foot, shin, and knee disorders, and it was not long before many podiatrists became heavily involved in the diagnosis and treatment of runners' injuries. We had believed for a long time that we could correct many of the problems by altering the mechanics of the runners' feet with an orthotic. We were also able to analyze the distinct wear patterns on the shoes of runners who had developed knee and other ailments.It was obvious to us that athletic footwear in those days left much to be desired, for it did little to help the runner compensate for any abnormalities in his gait. We also began to realize that the location of the pain and the cause of sports-related injuries were not always the same.

## Where Does It Hurt?

Pain is a hot area of research today, particularly the attempt to isolate the exact source of the pain and the relationship between that source and the parts of the body that hurt. For example, can knee pain be caused by a hip defect? Can abnormal biomechanics of the feet result in low back pain? We must remember that before this century very few medical experts related sciatica to low back abnormalities.

As a podiatrist who has devoted a lot of time to treating sports injuries, I have become acutely attuned to the relationships between foot problems and discomfort in other parts of the body.Therefore, I became directly involved in a fascinating study a few years ago at Mount Sinai Hospital in Toronto, the essence of which was to prove whether there were such relationships that could cause sciatic-type pain. The condition we were researching is called the piriformis syndrome, the existence of which is hotly disputed by some orthopedic specialists. Our studies strongly indicated a link between abnormal biomechanics of the feet and pain that mimicked sciatica, which is generally associated with low back problems. Our belief is based on the almost complete recovery of piriformis syndrome patients at the Sports Medicine Clinic at Mount Sinai Hospital after they had worn orthotics for three weeks. Our findings have now been verified by patient feedback, so we have every reason to believe that the condition does exist. We can also draw an analogy with that common problem of runners, chondromalacia patella (runner's knee). It often responds dramatically to footwear (with or without orthotics) that corrects a biomechanical foot problem. So there is solid evidence that the foot is indeed connected to the hip and the knee.

This illustrates my earlier point that people with musculoskeletal aches and pains, who have reason to suspect their feet are responsible for their woes, should try a good pair of running shoes for a couple of weeks. If your discomfort is significantly reduced, you know you are on the right track. You may achieve complete relief, or you may require an orthotic to fine-tune your biomechanics. In either case you will have avoided costly medical bills to treat painful disorders that could have been easily overcome with the help of new footwear.

This is not to say that you should first take your aching body to a shoe store rather than to your doctor. However, if medical opinion is that you have no serious illness, your next stop ought to be a store that carries good athletic footwear and has knowledgeable sales personnel. Shop before you drop; don't wait until your aching body cannot carry you one step farther!

## Common Overuse Syndromes

*Stressed Out*

Let's get to specifics, beginning with the forefront of the action. Forefoot injuries are as common today as they were in the last two decades, when runners and aerobic enthusiasts punished their feet mercilessly. However, one particular type of overuse injury is rapidly becoming more prevalent than the others—stress fractures of two types of bones, the metatarsals and the sesamoids. The difference between a stress fracture and other breaks is that the bone is not displaced. It simply "slices" in one place because of excess stress. X-rays will rarely pick up such a break, and the only way to isolate the exact location of the fracture is to do a bone scan. Stress fractures are more common today because of changing lifestyles. We have become more active, which is good, but we often wear improper shoes and overindulge in our physical labors, which is bad. The bones of our feet are constantly pounded by exposure to hard surfaces over which we walk, run, and jump, and it is the forefoot that often takes the brunt of the abuse. To illustrate, many years ago U.S. Marines in basic training were required to undertake twenty-mile runs in army boots, hardly the type of footwear one would want to wear for even a one-mile run. Regardless of their physical condition, these raw recruits often came down with metatarsal stress fractures, which became known as march breaks, a term that is used to this day.

The symptoms of a metatarsal stress fracture are

usually quite distinct. There is significant swelling initially on the top of the foot, and exquisite pain and tenderness directly above the break. An x-ray will not show the break for about four to six weeks, when healing is well under way. Since the symptoms are normally unique, I will not order a bone scan unless the patient is still in distress after about eight weeks. Why expose a person to an unnecessary dose of radiation?

The best thing to do with a stress fracture of a metatarsal bone is to leave it alone to heal by itself. Naturally, the injured person will have to be careful not damage or irritate the area further, so strenuous activities and long walks are out of the question until the bone has healed. Ice will help initially, but there is no need either to cast or to bandage the foot during the healing process. Once the pain and swelling have subsided, the person can resume a fairly normal lifestyle—minus the exercising! Women should not wear high-heels during the recovery period, which is approximately eight to twelve weeks.

Sesamoid bone stress fractures are not as easy to diagnose and treat as metatarsal breaks. Broken sesamoids do not heal easily; they are chunky pieces of bone, and the blood supply to the area is poor, which hinders healing. Moreover, the bones lie within major tendons on the bottom of the foot. As a person walks these tendons pull on the sesamoids, which creates more inflammation, pain, and increased separation of the fractured pieces of bone.

A fractured sesamoid bone will rarely unite completely. However, it may heal sufficiently so that all symptoms will eventually disappear. Recovery time will depend on the patient's ability to rest the foot sufficiently to allow healing to continue unimpeded.

There are three medical ways to approach such a fracture. The first is to let the foot heal by itself. After a few weeks a partial fusion of the bone should have naturally occurred, and the area should become symptom-free. Occasionally, the healing process can be helped with an orthotic, which ensures that there is no abnormal stress on the bone when the patient is walking. If the sesamoid bone refuses to heal normally, and if the patient is suffering constant discomfort, option number three is surgical removal of the fractured bone. If the operation is properly done, there is very little long-term effect on the patient's biomechanics, and the affected area returns to normal after a brief recovery period.

### Right in the Middle

Stress fractures in the midfoot used to be a rarity. The bones are larger, more stable, and not as prone to injury as bones in the forefoot or the rearfoot. How times have changed. I have seen ten stress fractures in the mid-tarsal region in the past eighteen months, and all were caused by overuse.

Let me give you an example of a typical midfoot fracture. I have a young cousin who is a rock guitarist and an avid runner. He was constantly pounding on his feet—running, racing from gig to gig with his musical equipment on his back, and tapping his feet while he rehearsed or played concerts. Eventually his instep began to hurt, particularly when he was tapping his toes while playing. This seriously affected his ability to perform well. He went to three doctors and had x-rays taken of his sore foot, all of which were negative. Finally he hobbled into my office in great distress, each painful stride aided by a cane. I carefully examined his foot and took down the history of his complaint. I determined that he had suffered a stress fracture of one of the three cuneiform bones in his midfoot. My diagnosis was confirmed a few days later by a bone scan. It was obvious that the stress of constantly running, walking, and toe-tapping had so weakened the affected bone that it eventually cracked.

Because the cuneiform bones are large, they take time to heal. Assuming that stress fractures of bones in the foot are caused solely by overuse and have no underlying organic foundation, they normally heal on their own, without medical intervention. The recovery period varies with the size and location of the bone.

In my cousin's case, I suggested that he rest the foot as much as possible until his discomfort completely disappeared. I also recommended that he change his style of guitar playing. He followed my advice and was back to normal in a few weeks.

We are now seeing stress fractures and other overuse syndromes that were rare only a few years ago. While we have certainly become more health-conscious, we have yet to adopt the sensible lifestyles that would enable us to avoid such problems.

### Winning Your Spurs

A few years ago overuse syndromes affecting the rearfoot were most often caused by sports injuries. Unhappily, this is no longer the case. The most common rearfoot condition, plantar fasciitis, is now just as prevalent in the general population because of improper footwear and a more active lifestyle. The condition is exacerbated by the fact that the longer we abuse our feet, the more likely we are to develop a pronation problem. The overuse syndrome leads to biomechanical abnormalities, which is essentially a reversal of the cause-and-effect relationship between lower limb dysfunction and abnormal biomechanics. In athletes, plantar fasciitis is most common in those who engage in activities that require constant side-to-side motion. Racquet sports are the major culprits; it is not unusual to find tennis or squash players with the disorder.The reason is the repeated, sudden lateral movements, which place tremendous torque-like stresses on the entire foot.

The distinctive symptoms of plantar fasciitis are acute pain in the middle and inside rear of the heel first thing in the morning and after prolonged sitting.There is no discoloration and usually no swelling.If swelling does occur it is minimal. Even though the symptoms are tell-tale, the condition is often misdiagnosed and too frequently x-rayed. It is not uncommon for patients to limp into my office, x-rays in hand, and announce that they are suffering from heel spurs. The diagnosis had been made by an uninformed medical practitioner who requires a primer in orthopedics.

To illustrate the lack of knowledge among many of my peers, let me tell you about a recent patient of mine, a physician who had examined the x-rays of his own foot and determined that he had a heel spur, which was causing him his discomfort.I told him that heel spurs do not cause pain, and continued with a detailed explanation of the causes and symptoms of plantar fasciitis.

When I first wrote about plantar fasciitis, the consensus was that the excruciating pain was caused by an inflammation and tearing of the ligaments (plantar fasciae) that attach the heel bone to the five metatarsal bones. Abnormal pronation was, and still is, considered the primary factor in the development of this condition. However, we have recently discovered that the problem is not a "flattening" of the foot—an over-stretching of the fasciae—but a powerful torque action that dramatically shortens the fasciae by twisting them tightly. Moreover, the pain is located not in the fasciae but in the lining (periosteum) of the bones from which the fasciae are being pulled away. The periosteum provides an attaching surface for bone and soft tissue, such as muscles, tendons, and ligaments. The twisted plantar fasciae are tearing that lining away from the bone, which itself has no nerve endings, so cannot feel pain. The periosteum, though, is loaded with ultrasensitive nerve endings, and when it is ripped away from its bone, it hurts terribly. The condition is known as periostitis.

Abnormal pronation leads to the devastating torque action that causes the plantar fasciae to twist and pull away from the bones, most commonly the heel bone. In this case the heel does not pronate sufficiently when the foot first strikes the ground, and the forefoot over-pronates when it comes in contact with the ground. These two abnormalities create the torquing action in the midfoot, which, in turn, causes the plantar fasciae to twist and, therefore, shorten. The condition can be compared to the elbow injuries commonly incurred by tennis players and baseball pitchers who try to throw a lot of curves. Different parts of the arm are subjected to abnormal torquing motions required to hit tennis shots or throw curve balls, and the soft tissue connected to bones at the elbow joint becomes twisted. It then pulls away from the bones, causing such injuries as tennis elbow.

When soft tissue tears away from bone, the affected bone will "chase" after the tissue to reattach itself. However, as long as the causes of the problem remain, it cannot catch up. But it continues to produce excessive osteoblast activity, which promotes growth of bone. So the bone lengthens, and if we eventually examine the area with x-rays we see "spurs," or bone extensions. The new bone resembles a ridge or a shelf, rather than a spur.) If we were to take a bone scan of the affected site when the condition first flares, we would pick up this increased osteoblast activity. Such activity is usually associated with a bone fracture, so we must be careful not to misdiagnose the problem as one of a broken heel. Heel bones rarely break; only a severe trauma, such as a fall from a great height that is broken by the feet, could cause a heel fracture. Foot specialists should not make that mistake, because the symptoms of plantar fasciitis are so characteristic.

I explained all this to my physician patient, but he remained convinced that he was suffering from a bone disorder, namely heel spurs. The conversation was reaching a stalemate when Dr. Hamilton Hall, the noted orthopod and back specialist, walked by the examining room. (Dr. Hall and I share office space.) I asked him to intercede to break the deadlock, and he listened to my patient explain his diagnosis.

"A spur is bone," Dr. Hall said, "and bones do not have nerve endings, so they can't hurt." End of argument. The physician was now willing to listen to my reasoning, having yielded to a higher god. In fact, the only time a bone spur can cause pain is when, in rare cases, it begins to press on a nerve, a condition that can occur in the back.

The symptoms of plantar fasciitis—excruciating pain in the morning upon arising, and after the victim has been sitting in one place for a long time and then bears weight—appear to indicate that the body is trying to heal itself when there is no weight on the affected foot. The plantar fasciae are not being twisted and shortened, and the periosteum is attempting to reattach itself to the bone. But when people with plantar fasciitis get back on their feet after a long resting period, all the good work is undone. The partially reattached lining is again ripped away from the bone, which causes the initial bout of exquisite pain. The pain may continue throughout the day, but will seem less acute.

Considering the sensitivity of the inflamed area, and the constant opportunities for reinjuring it, how can we cure plantar fasciitis and prevent it from recurring? Prevention is obviously the first choice of action. We can now see with our computer gait analysis equipment how under-pronation of the rearfoot combined with over-pronation of the forefoot produces tremendous torque action on the plantar fasciae. So we are able to identify the risk of plantar fasciitis before it occurs, or when it is quite mild, and correct the abnormal biomechanics with an orthotic.Wearing proper shoes will also help eliminate abnormal pronation.

If the inflammation caused by plantar fasciitis has become severe, we may have to treat the condition more aggressively. Although I hate to prescribe anti-inflammatory drugs because of their potential side effects, they may occasionally be required when the condition is extremely painful. However, I will use only a non-steroid anti-inflammatory. The one form of physiotherapy that seems to work well is laser therapy, which has replaced ultrasound as the physiotherapy treatment of choice for plantar fasciitis. (I am not referring here to laser surgery, but to laser therapy.) Any form of aggressive treatment must be accompanied by a solution to the biomechanical fault that caused the problem in the first place. Therefore, a person who has developed plantar fasciitis must wear good shoes and an orthotic to prevent the condition from either becoming worse or recurring.

Recovery time for plantar fasciitis will depend on its severity. If the condition is mild, the patient should be relatively symptom-free within a few weeks, providing proper footwear and orthotics are worn. If the inflammation is more acute, recovery may take up to three months, and perhaps longer if the problem has existed for a long time without being properly treated. Once healing is complete—when the periosteum has reattached to the bone—the discomfort should disappear altogether. In the final stages of recovery there may still be some discomfort first thing in the morning. Not to worry, though. That pain will eventually disappear as well, and is not an indication by itself of a recurrence of the disorder.

Unfortunately, not all cases of plantar fasciitis will respond to non-surgical treatments. One of my patients is a thirty-year-old-woman, Mary, who suffered with the disorder for almost one year before being operated on to repair the damage. When she first came to me in October 1989, Mary was complaining of swelling in the ankle area and on top of the foot. The pain in her heel was excruciating. She agreed with my advice to obtain a pair of custom-made orthotics to correct the over-pronation that was causing her problem. Because it takes a while for the orthotics to make a difference, and because she was in severe pain, I also prescribed an anti-inflammatory drug.

The orthotics and anti-inflammatory medication did not help. By December, Mary was in such agony that, at times, she was forced to crawl on the floor because she could not put any weight on her feet. I prescribed different anti-inflammatory medication for her and ordered a different style of orthotics. The new treatment was equally unsuccessful.

In January 1990 I referred Mary to an orthopedic surgeon. He agreed that she was suffering from plantar fasciitis and gave her a third anti-inflammatory drug. He also did some blood tests and, subsequently, sent her to see a rheumatologist. The final diagnosis was the same as the original one—plantar fasciitis. Mary was now describing her symptoms in the following manner.

"Every step I took felt like I was walking over a golf ball," she said. "When the pain became unbearable it would run up my leg to the knee area and give a burning sensation. In the morning when I first got out of bed I would have to limp to the shower. In the evening when sitting down the pain would return as the plantar fasciae were trying to heal."

The orthopedic surgeon advised Mary to stay off her feet as much as possible, and to lose weight, which would help relieve some of the pressure on her feet. She went on to lose quite a bit of weight, but the pain persisted. Moreover, the discomfort spread to one hip and her previously unaffected left foot. At this point I tried cortisone injections into the inflamed area. After the second shot failed to help I had her return to the orthopedic surgeon.It was decided that surgery was the only remaining option because the plantar fasciae had obviously been so damaged that non-invasive treatments were insufficient.In all my years of podiatric practice I can count on the fingers of one hand all the plantar fasciitis patients who have required surgery.

The "plantar release" surgery was performed in July 1990. It involves cutting the plantar fasciae to allow them to reattach properly to the calcaneus (heel) and metatarsal bones. Mary was required to use crutches and special "cast boots" while the area healed and the cut ends of the plantar fasciae joined together again. In September she was able to walk unaided, though in running shoes with new custom-made orthotics. Since she began wearing her new shoes and inserts the pain in her good foot has subsided dramatically, and her surgery healed normally by the end of the year. Because the incision was made on the side of her foot, not on the bottom, she will not have any problems from scar tissue on weight-bearing parts of the foot. Her plantar fasciitis problems should not recur.

## Without a Good Leg to Stand On

A host of other lower limb problems are, like plantar fasciitis, caused by a shortening of ligaments due to abnormal pronation.The most commonly diagnosed of these conditions are Achilles tendinitis and chondromalacia patella, or runner's knee. Let's focus on these two disorders, then move up the leg until we reach the lower back.

### Achilles Tendinitis

For many years people with this condition were regularly

treated improperly with heel lifts—a quarter to half an inch—which were thought to reduce the strain on the Achilles tendon. Medical practitioners did not understand the biomechanical dysfunctions that most often cause the problem, although they recognized that the tendon was too short. The heel lifts were an attempt to bridge the gap between the heel bone (calcaneus) and the lower leg. In fact, the lifts were allowing the Achilles tendon to shorten even more, which is not a long-term solution to the problem (see Diagram 9).

Achilles tendinitis develops for two reasons: the tendon is gradually shortened by the constant wearing of high-heeled shoes, or abnormal pronation is causing it to twist and therefore shorten. As with other leg and foot problems, Achilles tendinitis used to be primarily a concern of athletes. It is now a common overuse syndrome that cuts a wide swath across the population, which has become more physically active in the past few years but is still quite naive about proper foot care.

In Chapter Four I noted that a typical Achilles tendinitis sufferer is a woman who has been inactive for many years and who has been regularly wearing high-heeled shoes socially and to work. Her Achilles tendon has shortened, and when she decides to undertake an exercise program, she fails to incorporate the proper stretching routine into her warm-up exercises. As a result the Achilles tendon is over-stretched and begins to pull away from the calcaneus, the lining of which tears away from the bone. The pain the woman begins to experience is from calcaneal periostitis, the same type of disorder as plantar fasciitis. If the inflammation is not too severe, and the woman does not have a biomechanical fault, she should recover nicely in

*Diagram 9*
**The Achilles Tendon**

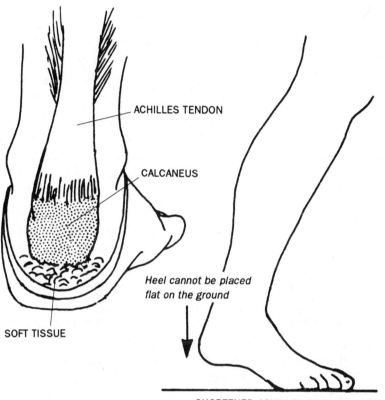

ACHILLES TENDON

CALCANEUS

*Heel cannot be placed flat on the ground*

SOFT TISSUE

SHORTENED ACHILLES TENDON

a few weeks with a bit of physiotherapy and proper stretching exercises. She must also realize that, when she returns to an exercise regimen, she must continue to stretch the tendon at the beginning and end of her workout to avoid a recurrence of the problem. Naturally, it would help if she began wearing lower-heeled shoes regularly.

The other major cause of Achilles tendinitis is abnormal pronation, which affects men and women equally. The Achilles tendon is attached at the bottom to the calcaneus and at the top to the calf muscle, which in turn is attached to the femur (the thigh bone) just above the knee. The Achilles tendon is extremely important, because the whole leg acts as a single unit when we walk. So, when the foot first strikes the ground and begins to pronate naturally, the leg follows suit. When the foot reaches mid-stance and then starts lifting off the ground, it goes through a brief neutral stage before normal supination occurs. The rest of the leg also naturally follows the same range of motions. In the pronation phase, the leg is said to rotate internally; during supination, it rotates externally. If abnormal pronation occurs during any stage of the gait cycle, the lower leg will behave similarly. However, the upper part of the leg is usually unable to follow the same abnormal rotation. Therefore, the Achilles tendon is being pulled one way at the top and in the opposite direction at the bottom, so it then twists and becomes shorter. The weakest point of the tendon is at the heel bone, and it begins to pull away from the calcaneal periosteum. As we now know, the result is Achilles tendinitis.

If the primary cause of Achilles tendinitis is abnormal pronation, neither stretching exercises nor physiotherapy will help, because the biomechanical fault will remain. So any treatment must include a correction of the abnormal pronation that caused the inflammation. The course of action is to wear proper footwear with prescribed orthotic inserts.

One of my patients, George, is an active fifty-six-year-old who came down with Achilles tendinitis about ten years ago. He had been an enthusiastic runner for many years and was not content to follow the advice of doctors who told him that "those ankles and knees are not made for jogging any more."

George had been competing in a number of 10-kilometer races when "boom, it suddenly happened—dull, searing pain at the top of the heel." He limped into one clinic and, after being examined, was told that he should have his heels surgically scraped to remove the calcium buildup. He thought this to be a rather drastic measure and went to the Sports Medicine Clinic at Mount Sinai Hospital in Toronto, where I first met him.

After watching George walk for a few minutes I determined that his Achilles tendinitis would probably respond well with orthotics. I advised him not to have his heels scraped. George immediately ordered his inserts and was running again in six weeks.

George has been wearing orthotics ever since, in his running and dress shoes, and continues to run up to three miles every day. I see him every two years, when he comes in for a re-evaluation and new orthotics. In the past ten years he has had occasional twinges of pain in the Achilles tendon area, but requires nothing more than ice to relieve the symptoms.

### Chondromalacia Patella

The common term for this unpleasant malady is runner's knee, because it is so closely associated with the running and jogging craze that began two decades ago.

Chondromalacia patella (which basically translates as a softening of the cartilage in the kneecap) is caused in the same manner as plantar fasciitis and Achilles tendinitis.In this case abnormal pronation forces the patellar tendon to be pulled to the inside by the internal rotation of the lower leg. At the same time, the external rotation of the upper part of the leg is twisting the knee joint to the outside. The kneecap (patella) normally moves up and down within a groove that lies between the medial and lateral femoral condyles (rounded protuberances at the end of the femur bone). The external rotation of the femur simultaneous with the internal rotation of the patellar tendon yanks the patella out of its normal track between the condyles. The patella begins rubbing on the condyles, and the cartilage on the back of the patella is subjected to severely abnormal wear and tear.

The most common symptoms of chondromalacia patella are acute pain radiating from the top of the kneecap—particularly when walking up or down stairs—and stiffness in the joint after two or more hours of sitting with a bent leg and then bearing weight. Also, mobility of the knee joint is affected, so that the normal range of motions is restricted.

In most cases, a program to treat and cure the problem will most likely include orthotics to eliminate the abnormal pronation.Physiotherapy to relieve the inflammation and build up the muscles in the leg may be required. Surgery is necessary only if the condition has been allowed to progress to the point where the knee joint has become severely damaged because the cartilage has almost completely worn out and bone is grinding against bone. A few years ago a technique was developed by an orthopedic surgeon whereby a piece of human or bovine bone is wedged under the patellar tendon. This procedure lifts the kneecap completely off the knee joint, which prevents the pain caused by bones rubbing together. It has been quite successful so far, although more time is probably needed to determine its long-term effectiveness. The only side effect to date has been the appearance of an extra-small bump just below the knee—a small price to pay for relief from debilitating pain.

One other cause of chondromalacia patella is growing pains. Young girls—usually in their teens—may develop the condition for two reasons. Firstly, they tend not to grow evenly, particularly in the area of their hips, which often results in abnormal biomechanics until everything is finally in synch. Secondly, they begin experimenting with fashion footwear and may end up wearing shoes—particularly high-heeled ones—that adversely affect their biomechanics. The condition usually resolves itself with a minimum of intervention once they are fully grown, and if they avoid improper footwear. Occasionally, physiotherapy and a proper exercise program may be required if the inflammation has become severe.

### A Kick on the Shins

You can now see how a simple biomechanical foot fault can lead to an inflammation of the knee joint and cause problems in the ankle area. Well, overuse injuries can also develop in between those two trouble spots. The most common of these are shin splints.

A shin splint is basically our old friend periostitis, in a different location. There are two variations of the disorder, the medial or tibialis posterior and the lateral or tibialis anterior, depending on where the periosteum is being torn away from the tibia and by which muscle in the leg (see Diagram 10).

*Diagram 10*
**Anterior and Posterior Sites of Splints**

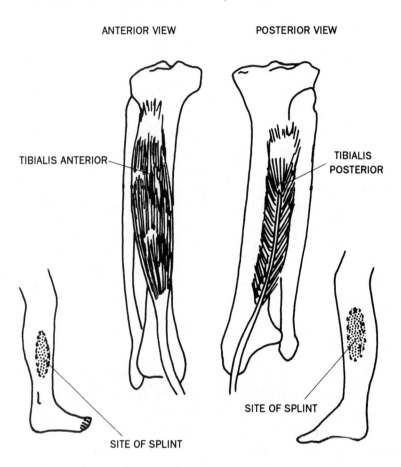

ANTERIOR VIEW          POSTERIOR VIEW

TIBIALIS ANTERIOR

TIBIALIS
POSTERIOR

SITE OF SPLINT

SITE OF SPLINT

The tibialis posterior muscle runs down the inside of the leg from the tibia to the bottom of the foot. Its tendon attaches at the bottom to the base of the first four metatarsal bones.It is a major anti-pronating muscle— that is, it helps prevent the lower leg and foot from over-pronating.Unfortunately, when there is abnormal pronation in the rear part of the foot, the "tib post" muscle and tendon can become overworked. This can occur when a person who overpronates engages in a form of exercise that places undue stress on the legs and feet, such as running or high-impact aerobics.When the tib post muscle is overused, it becomes "tight." Tendons are then forced to stretch abnormally to keep it from tearing. Since the attachment of a tendon to its muscle is stronger than its attachment to bone, the tib post tendon begins to pull away from the tibia. The periosteum then tears away from the tibia.The result is painful periostitis. In sports medicine circles the condition is known as a shin splint. As with other types of periostitis, a bone scan of the area will probably give a false reading of a stress fracture. Therefore, it is imperative that an active person with acute pain and extreme tenderness in the lower part of the leg seek help from an expert in sports-related injuries; otherwise oper treatment may be given.

If a tibialis posterior syndrome is left untreated, and the person continues to overuse the leg, the tib post tendon may eventually rupture. When this occurs the affected foot completely flattens, the person over-pronates violently and appears to be walking on the ankle bone. As one might expect, the rupturing of the tendon can produce intense discomfort. Unfortunately, it will never heal completely by itself; nor can it be resewn. If the pain remains unbearable it may be necessary in the long term to "fuse" the ankle— that is, join the ankle bones together to stabilize the area. This procedure will prevent the foot from over-pronating but will also eliminate the ankle joint's normal range of motions. Such surgery is a last resort; the logical approach would be to prevent such an injury from occurring in the first place.

The second type of shin splint is the anterior, or tibialis anterior. The "tib ant" muscle runs down the outside of the leg and foot from the tibia to the metatarsal bones (see Diagram 11). Like the tibialis posterior, it is also an anti-pronation muscle that can be adversely affected by abnormal forefoot pronation. However, it is more common for anterior shin splints to be caused by the muscle itself, rather than primarily by a foot problem. The periostitis occurs on the outside rather than the inside part of the leg.

Prevention is the best way to avoid shin splints, which, if left untreated once they occur, can lead to stress fractures of either the tibia or the fibula, or, as I mentioned, a ruptured tendon. If they do develop, rest, ice, and ultrasound therapy will relieve the symptoms. Obviously, elimination of the cause of the condition must follow to ensure that it does not recur. Sensible exercise regimens—including stretching properly—combined with the wearing of good athletic shoes and orthotics to prevent abnormal pronation should prevent further episodes of the shin splints.

Shin splints and ruptured tib post tendons are far too common, and can easily be avoided. There are many types of aerobic exercises that do not place as much stress on the tibialis posterior and anterior muscles as running and high-impact aerobics. Most important, you must forget the silly notion that there is no gain without pain. If your legs start to hurt while you are exercising, stop immediately. Your body is telling you that something is amiss, not that you need to increase your pain-tolerance levels.

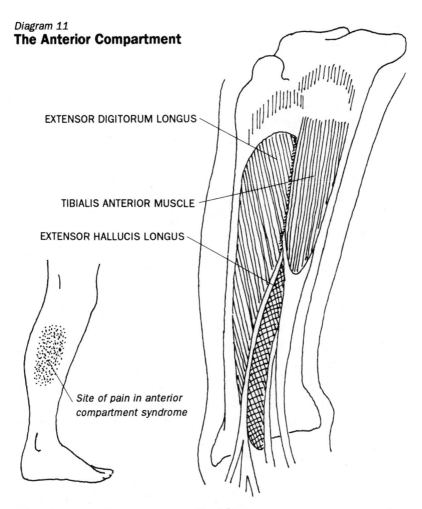

*Diagram 11*
**The Anterior Compartment**

EXTENSOR DIGITORUM LONGUS

TIBIALIS ANTERIOR MUSCLE

EXTENSOR HALLUCIS LONGUS

*Site of pain in anterior compartment syndrome*

*The Anterior Compartment Syndrome*

This syndrome is slightly more exotic than the others discussed in this chapter, but because it can become an acute problem it is well worth mentioning.The anterior compartment is the front part of the lower leg. Many muscles pass through this area, and there are small compartments between them (see Diagram 11). If one or more of the muscles becomes inflamed, there is increased pressure within the compartments, which can cause pinching of the blood vessels and reduced blood flow to the region. This may lead to mild discomfort, which is often mistaken for shin splints. This is as serious as the syndrome gets in most cases, and it can be treated with rest, ice, and physiotherapy. The cause is almost always a combination of abnormal biomechanics and improper exercising—insufficient warm-up, stretching, and cool-down routines.

On rare occasions a severe injury in the area of the anterior compartment will require immediate medical attention. Last summer a major league baseball player was running when he tripped rounding first base. He immediately felt a burning sensation deep in one lower leg. As the game wore on the leg became increasingly swollen, to the point where he could hardly put any weight on it. The trainer's alert judgment and response probably saved the player from serious long-term leg problems.

When the ball player injured his leg he suffered internal bleeding in the anterior compartment. This resulted in two to three times the normal amount of pressure in the compartment, which caused extreme swelling and pain. The athlete was taken to hospital, where surgery was performed to relieve the pressure in the compartment and to repair the muscle and blood vessel tears that had caused the bleeding. The ball player made a rapid recovery after the surgery and missed only one month of the season.

Now, you don't have to trip over first base to develop an acute anterior compartment syndrome. You could stumble on the sidewalk or in your own home and give yourself an equally nasty injury. However, you may take comfort in knowing that such an acute trauma is a rare occurrence.

### The Piriformis Syndrome

I mentioned at the beginning of this chapter that one of our projects at the Sports Medicine Clinic at Toronto's Mount Sinai Hospital is the search for the elusive and controversial piriformis syndrome.

The sciatic nerve is the aggrieved party in this overuse condition. This nerve runs down from the spine through the leg. For years sciatica was thought to be caused solely by a pinched sciatic nerve in the lower back. The three causes of this impingement (pinching) are a herniated lumbar disc, a facet-joint abnormality, and a narrowing of the spinal canal through which the nerve must pass.

My colleagues and I strongly believe that the sciatic nerve can, in fact, be pinched in the upper part of the leg where it passes under the piriformis muscle (see Diagram 12). One function of this muscle is to prevent the femur from over-rotating to compensate for abnormal pronation in the foot.

When the foot over-pronates, the lower leg follows suit but the upper leg does not. This produces a torsion action on various muscles and tendons, the result of which may be Achilles tendinitis, chondromalacia patella, and other disorders. Occasionally the upper part of the leg will also over-pronate, and this action contorts the piriformis muscle, which then pinches the sciatic nerve. This is only a simple explanation of the syndrome. The biomechanics are extremely complicated and the theory quite controversial.

Thanks to the development of video gait analysis, equip-

*Diagram 12*
**Sciatic Nerve and Piriformis Syndrome**

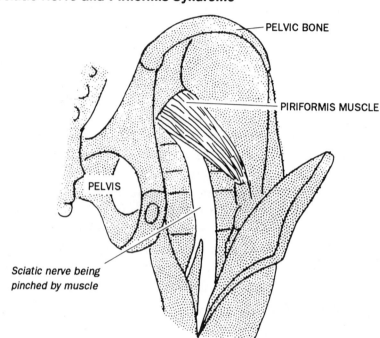

PELVIC BONE

PIRIFORMIS MUSCLE

PELVIS

*Sciatic nerve being
pinched by muscle*

ment, we can now observe how the motions of the foot can affect the rolling of the hips. Unfortunately, we are usually unable to pinpoint precisely how and where the piriformis muscle is pinching the sciatic nerve. The state-of-the-art diagnostic equipment for determining such findings is the MRI or the CAT scanner. The machines are very expensive to operate and are normally available only for much more serious ailments. I assume that newer, less costly, more readily available equipment will soon enable us to routinely isolate and accurately measure the site of these nerve impingements.

Since the sciatic-type pain associated with the piriformis syndrome usually disappears within a month after orthotics are worn, there is no reason to prescribe any other form of treatment. If, however, the pain persists, the condition may be primarily one of a low back dysfunction, in which case more diagnostic tests are indicated.

### Oh, My Aching Back

In Chapter One I related the story of the patient who experienced almost instant relief from her back pain after she put inserts into her shoes. She is not the only person whose low back pain was greatly reduced or eliminated by orthotics. Unfortunately, her reaction is not quite the norm; I would be hard pressed to argue that orthotics alone can cure all types of back ailments.

Although most medical experts agree that there can be a strong connection between abnormal biomechanics and low back discomfort, the relationships are still difficult to establish and to understand. We can observe, with the aid of sophisticated video and computer equipment, how abnormal pronation in the foot can affect the leg right up to the hip. But we are still unable to dissect the biomechanics of the spinal column when a person walks. I can only assume that a relationship does indeed exist between foot and back disorders because some of my patients experience fairly rapid relief from back pain after wearing orthotics.

One of my theories is that when people walk abnormally to the point of causing themselves foot or other lower limb pain, they subconsciously alter their gait to eliminate the discomfort. When this happens their gait becomes even more abnormal, so they begin placing undue stress on joints and soft tissue (muscles, tendons, ligaments) in their upper legs and hips. The hip is connected to the lower back at the top and to the upper leg at the bottom. If we walk abnormally, we may eventually produce abnormal wear and tear on the hip joint and surrounding tissues. Anyone who has experienced pain in the hips will know that it may force a person to walk abnormally in an effort to avoid the discomfort. However, this new gait will produce even worse biomechanics, which results in a pulling and twisting of soft tissue masses that are connected to the hips and the lower back. Hence, the onset of low back pain.

The above scenario is all too common, but easily preventable. If a person who has foot or leg pain caused by abnormal biomechanics receives swift and proper treatment, the problems should never spread higher up to the hip and lower back. One of my patients is typical of what happens when a biomechanical fault, combined with an overuse syndrome caused by a new physical activity, resulted in a chronic back problem.

Sue is an active forty-two-year-old who has suffered various aches and pains since she undertook a more strenuous exercise program seven years ago. When she was thirty-five she began taking aerobics classes.Before that her physical activities were confined to long, brisk walks and swimming. She had no idea at that time about the importance of wearing proper athletic shoes when doing aerobics, and within two years she had developed lower back problems. She began twice-weekly sessions with a chiropractor, and her back gradually improved.Then she developed an ankle injury, which prompted her chiropractor to suggest that she see me.

Sue had a host of biomechanical problems. Her hips turned out, she was somewhat knock-kneed and toed-out when she walked, and she badly over-pronated. I prescribed custom-made orthotics for her, and she continued receiving chiropractic treatments. Her lower back improved, but her ankle did not respond sufficiently to avoid more aggressive action.

Sue was seen by a doctor who specializes in sports medicine. He prescribed a series of ultrasound treatments and, as a final resort, cortisone injections into the ankle area to reduce the inflammation. There was no relief. The doctor then recommended an arthroscopy (minimal-incision surgery to inspect and repair the damaged area), which revealed an outgrowth of fibula bone that was irritating the ankle joint. The bone was shaved to prevent further inflammation of the joint. The operation was moderately successful: the severe ankle pain diminished greatly, but only when Sue wore her orthotics.

Sue claims that she can now wear regular shoes without orthotics for a short while but that she must wear them most of the time when exercising. I would prefer, of course, that she wear orthotics regularly, particularly since she has begun to develop a bunion, which appears to have a genetic cause. I recently prescribed new orthotics for her, which she wears in her running shoes and which have provided relief from the discomforts of her bunion and her lower back. However, she continues to suffer when wearing other shoes. To date I have been unable to convince her to wear fashion orthotics.

Sue is typical of the person who undertakes a new, rigorous exercise program without first ensuring that she is both physically and biomechanically sound. In her own words, "I cannot stress enough the importance of proper testing before embarking on new high-stress physical activities. If I had been tested, I would have discovered my potential problems before I was injured. I would have had orthotics from the beginning, my ankle would never have become weak enough to be injured, and I probably would not have had to undergo as much chiropractic treatment."

## Newer Exercise Fads

This section will cover some of the newer popular forms of exercise to help you determine whether they are suitable for you. Many of the recent fads are really not all that new; others are quite novel and attempt to reduce the likelihood of overuse syndromes so common in athletic endeavors that were popular in the 1980s, particularly running and high-impact aerobics.

### Stair-climbing Machines

The stair-climber has become popular recently because it produces low-impact aerobic activity—that is, there is no constant pounding on the lower extremities from running or jumping. So it can be an excellent way to improve cardiopulmonary fitness without unduly stressing the feet and legs.

However, stair-climbing dramatically increases the amount of stretching and pulling on the back of the legs. This results in increased stress on the knees and may produce chondromalacia patella. The irritation will only become worse if you continue to exercise on a stair-climber, because you are repeatedly standing on one leg for a biomechanically abnormal longer time with all the body weight behind the knee, rather than over it. This situation will be exacerbated in people who have chronically short Achilles tendons, which will be repeatedly stretched much farther than their capability. These people may develop Achilles tendinitis as well as chondromalacia patella.

The wear and tear caused by stair-climbing is quite different from that caused by constant pounding on the lower limbs from running or jumping exercises. Overuse syndromes such as shin splints are much rarer; also, there is far less impact on the knee joint itself.

If you choose stair-climbing as your exercise, you can lessen the risk of developing chondromalacia patella and Achilles tendinitis by properly stretching before you begin climbing. And you must be careful not to attempt breaking Guinness stair-climbing records before your lower limbs are ready for the challenge.

### Low-impact Aerobics

This type of aerobic exercise is far less stressful on the legs and feet than high-impact aerobics, which features a lot of jumping up and down. Since there is basically no jumping involved in low-impact aerobics, there is a significant decrease in the number of shin splints and stress fractures of the foot and lower leg. Also, the exercise routines are much easier for beginners, because they place less stress on most of the body. So a beginner can ease into the fitness program with less likelihood of a discouraging debilitating injury at the onset.

The one problem area for those doing low-impact aerobics is the Achilles tendon. As in stair-climbing, the entire foot is usually on the ground much longer than normal, so there is added stress on the back of the leg and foot. People with abnormally short Achilles tendons—particularly women who have worn high-heeled shoes regularly for years—may develop minor Achilles tendinitis unless they stretch properly before doing the exercise routines.

### Treadmills

The beauty of the treadmill is that people can run or walk normally on a constantly level surface in a controlled environment.They can also adjust the speed and incline of the treadmill according to their fitness levels.The advantage of running or walking on a consistently even surface is that there is less risk of taking a bad step—and thereby suffering an injury—or of creating an artificial biomechanical problem.The latter may occur for two reasons.

Firstly, people who train outdoors on the streets may be unknowingly running on canted surfaces. For example, streets are often slightly sloped to allow water to run off into sewers. Having one foot regularly landing lower than the other is akin to having one leg longer than the other. Severe biomechanical problems can result, particularly if the runner already pronates abnormally. Runners in this situation may develop a neuroma, which results from the heads of the metatarsal bones being squeezed together in the space between the toes.

Secondly, people who run regularly on indoor tracks are constantly negotiating narrow, tight corners, and often have to swerve to avoid other runners. This repeated sharp turning places tremendous stress on the ankle and knee joints and is often responsible for overuse syndromes in those areas.

If you only walk on the treadmill, there is no real

downside to the exercise.However, if you run on the machine, you are subjecting yourself to the same high-impact forces associated with the pounding caused by running on other types of surfaces.

*Rowing Machines and Cycling*
These forms of exercise are becoming more popular. As with other types of exercise equipment, you can control your own program and environment.Since they are basically non-weight-bearing activities, they are also appropriate for some people with lower limb problems. However, those with disc or facet joint problems in their backs or necks, or with severe knee problems, will have their conditions exacerbated by the heavy stress that rowing places on those parts of the body. Dr. Hamilton Hall, the best-selling author of two books on back disorders, suggests that anyone with such problems obtain expert medical advice before undertaking any exercise program.

Cyclists who have had knee problems should lower or raise the seat of their bicycle until they can ride without any discomfort both during and after exercising. I have one patient who began experiencing knee pain after purchasing a new stationary bicycle. Unfortunately, he bought a bike that did not have an adjustable seat, so he could not experiment with different heights. Cyclists who ride outdoors and wear special cycling shoes will find that adjusting the angle of the cleats on the shoes can also correct the mechanics of the cycling motion. If neither a different seat height nor a different cleat angle eliminates your knee pain, you should seek the help of a sports medicine expert.

*Triathlons and Cross-training*

When serious athletes began looking for new challenges, and ways to beat the overuse syndromes associated with long-distance running, they turned their attention to a combination of physical endeavors. The buzzwords today are triathlons and cross-training.

Triathletes who enter competitions are usually required to run 6 miles (10 km), cycle a marathon distance, and swim 1 mile (1.6 km). These distances may vary in different competitions. This sounds like a very masochistic, insane pastime, but there is a certain logic to the madness. There is far less wear and tear on weight-bearing parts of the body in a triathlon than in a marathon.

A marathoner runs more than 26 miles (42 km), often on uneven and hard terrain. And before the race he or she will accumulate hundreds of miles in training. Think of all that pounding on the lower limbs. Even a person with normal biomechanics will suffer some wear and tear in the hip, knee, ankle, and foot joints, and to the soft tissue masses in the legs and feet. This is why marathoners should limit the number of marathons they run each year so they can recuperate from the beating their bodies have taken during training and the race itself.

On the other hand, swimmers can retain their conditioning much more easily after competitions because they are not placing any undue stress on the weight-bearing parts of their bodies. Cyclists can also recover from long races more quickly than runners. Last summer I saw a cyclist being interviewed on television four days after he had completed the grueling Tour de France race. He claimed that he felt better at the end of the race than during its middle stages, and that he was in Toronto to compete in a 36-mile (60 km) race that weekend (which he won).

So there is good reason for the enthusiastic athlete to switch from marathon running to triathlons. The triathletes run only 6 miles (10 km) instead of 26 (42 km), and they reduce the stress on their lower limbs by swimming and cycling the remainder of the competition. Moreover, they do not have to run such long distances while in training. Triathletes are far less prone to overuse syndrome conditions than people who exercise by running long distances exclusively.

Cross-training is a less intensive way of exercising than competing in triathlons, but works on the same theory. The idea is to exercise all the muscle groups in the body while increasing cardiopulmonary fitness. The result is fewer overuse injuries and a more comprehensive training program for the entire body.

Cross-trainers will alternate days of running, aerobics, swimming, cycling, and other types of aerobic exercises with non-aerobic activities such as muscle toning, stretching, and body-building. For example, Monday may be running; Tuesday, swimming; Wednesday, the Universal gym; Thursday, aerobics; and so forth. By following such a routine, athletes can avoid overuse syndromes by giving parts of their bodies sufficient time to rest and recuperate from strenuous activity.

### Racquet Sports

During the 1970s and 1980s racquet sports clubs were the places to be, for both fitness and social activity. Squash and tennis players were regular visitors to my office and to the Sports Medicine Clinic at the Mount Sinai

Hospital. Although racquet sports are not quite as popular as they once were, there are still enough players around to keep me busy.

The major reason for foot and leg problems in racquet sport athletes is the enormous stress placed on the foot and ankle by the rapid stop-and-go and lateral movements required to chase and hit the ball. Also, tennis players place immense pressure on the sesamoid bones when they are serving, because so much of their body weight is on the area of the head of the first metatarsal as they stretch upwards to hit the ball.

Racquet sport players with biomechanical faults will exacerbate them with their movements on the court. As a result they may develop a whole range of foot problems, among them ankle sprains, Achilles tendinitis, plantar fasciitis, and sesamoiditis. To reduce the risk of such ailments, they must wear the proper shoes, preferably with orthotics, that will provide the feet with the required lateral support. As you will learn in the next chapter, squash and tennis shoes are designed and built to provide that support. Running shoes are not; they are designed for straight-ahead movements.

No doubt I have neglected to mention at least one physical activity in which you may be interested. If so, you can probably apply the information contained above to determine how best to avoid acute traumas or overuse syndromes. My advice is to shelve the notion of "no pain, no gain"; to wear the proper shoes, with corrective orthotics if you have a biomechanical fault that requires such intervention; and to know when to quit exercising for the day before you develop a problem.

# 8

# IF THE SHOE FITS...

IT WASN'T SO MANY YEARS AGO THAT A RUNNING shoe manufacturer produced footwear that tilted people to the outside part of their feet. The company put a five-degree wedge in the forefoot on the big toe side, which made the foot higher on the inside and lower on the outside and was an ill-conceived attempt to correct over-pronation. Although the concept worked for a few runners, many other unsuspecting purchasers with reasonably normal gaits were suddenly over-compensating and soon developed a wide variety of painful lower limb maladies.

A generation ago we also had the famous "negative heel" disaster.Two major shoe companies theorized that altogether too much weight was being borne by the ball of the foot.This could be corrected, they concluded, by designing a negative-heel shoe, placing the heel of the shoe lower than the sole, which altered the natural human gait by putting more weight at all times on the heel of the foot.They believed that their shoes would eliminate forever all forefoot problems, since the front part of the foot would no longer be subjected to excess stress.The shoes made a complete mess of the wearers' biomechanics and created a host of lower back and hip problems.Fortunately, negative-heel shoes and their negative results quickly disappeared.

Shoe manufacturers have come a long way since those early days of trial and error. In fact, the makers of athletic shoes are now in the forefront of a technological revolution that is attempting to produce the ultimate in footwear style, function, and comfort. I am truly amazed at the progress the shoe industry has made in the past five years. Two of the largest manufacturers have been spending well over $1 million a year in research in an attempt to understand the footwear needs of athletes and other active individuals. As I mentioned at the beginning of the book, about 90 per cent of the running shoes sold today are being purchased by non-runners who find them much more comfortable than other types of footwear.

## A Very Brief History of Shoemaking

A book on footwear manufacturing that appeared almost thirty years ago listed five basic purposes for shoes:

1. Protection from the elements, unfriendly beasties and man-made objects;
2. To assist in the performance of abnormal tasks, such as sports and work-related activities;
3. To overcome foot abnormalities;
4. To complete a "costume"; and
5. To indicate rank or office.

The author forgot one function of women's footwear, which has been obvious for centuries: to appeal to the more prurient instincts of men with foot fetishes or with an eye for a shapely calf. There are also indications throughout the ages, and even into this century, that men in some societies preferred women's shoes to be so uncomfortable as to keep them from walking far enough to get into mischief.

Therefore, while men's footwear has been reasonably comfortable for centuries, the same cannot be said for women's shoes. And although shoes for both sexes have provided at least a modicum of protection, they have only recently been designed to overcome foot abnormalities. Moreover, until the athletic shoe industry got its act together a few years ago, footwear did not adequately assist in performing "abnormal" tasks.

Until the seventeenth century, when English manufacturers began mass-producing army boots using manual labor, all shoes were made according to individual specifications by shoemakers. These craftsmen were held in high esteem in their communities, although they were not that well remunerated for their labors. It was not until the middle of the nineteenth century that hand tools were

replaced by machinery and production lines. So, from that
time on, only those who could afford the finest hand-
crafted footwear were able to have shoes and boots made
to fit their feet perfectly. However, these hand-made shoes
were not necessarily biomechanically sound. Only in the
latter half of the last century were shoes made specifically
for the left and the right foot. Before that all footwear was
straight-lasted—that is, no account was made for the
natural curvature of the two feet (a situation that still sadly
exists in the ballet world). To complicate matters, it was
only in the 1880s that sizes (full and half) were introduced
in England and North America.Therefore, it was quite
difficult until then to shop for shoes that fitted properly.

Women had an even more difficult time in the good old
days.Their plight has not changed that much over the
years, but at least they have the option today of purchasing
footwear that won't ruin their feet, legs, knees, and lower
back.

The two major problems with women's footwear seem
always to have  been excessively elevated heels and tight
toe-boxes.In sixteenth-century Venice, heels were often
so high that women needed the help of a maid or escort
to be able to walk at all. One pair of shoes from that era has
been preserved in a museum; it has heels over two feet
high.Yet none of the shoes in the museum over nine
inches high show any significant wear. One theory is that
the style came from Turkey, where women who lived in
the sultans' harems never walked very far. Fortunately,
shoes did not aspire to such great heights again until the
1950s, when the stiletto heel became the vogue. In fact, at
times in Europe and North America until the twentieth
century, shoes with exaggerated high heels were often

associated with wanton women. So only women of questionable morals wore them, unless they were intentionally trying to make a statement.

Men have also succumbed occasionally to the desire to be taller. In ancient Greece actors regularly wore three- to four-inch platform heels, made of cork, so that they could stand out on stage. Louis XIV of France, who reigned in the late 1600s, was quite short and very vain. He wore high-heeled shoes to increase his stature, and the style became the rage for aristocratic men of his day. Some of the heels were as high as five inches.

While women were thought to be sexier when they wore high heels, they were also often considered desirable if they had tiny feet that could squeeze into even smaller shoes. We have all heard about the old Chinese custom of binding the feet of young girls so that they had lilliputian feet when they grew up and were able to walk only with a gait that men considered sensuous. In parts of Europe and North America in the mid-1800s, after anesthetics were invented, some women actually had one or two toes amputated so that they would have smaller, sexier feet that could fit into the very narrow shoes so common then.

In the late 1800s North American women, who tended to walk much more than European women, were becoming quite interested in comfort. As a result, by the turn of the century shoes were available in a variety of sizes and widths in the New World. However, it was still far too early in the game for shoe designers and manufacturers to understand clearly the dynamics of the human gait. Therefore, the relationship between the biomechanics of walking and foot and lower limb problems remained basically undiscovered.

One man did attempt a rudimentary study of the dynamic forces on the feet when a person was walking or running, and he became a household name—Salvatore Ferragamo.When he emigrated to the United States in 1914 he was appalled by the lack of comfort in women's footwear, so he set out to produce comfortable, stylish shoes. Ferragamo may have been the first shoemaker to appreciate what happened to a foot when it was squashed into a shoe that was much too narrow. Unfortunately, he was unable to appreciate how a higher heel could also adversely affect the foot. So what he produced was a high-heeled shoe with a wider toe-box and a solid steel arch support to enhance the wearer's comfort.His shoes became a big hit in Hollywood in the 1920s, yet he returned to Italy in 1927 because he could not find enough skilled craftsmen in the United States to meet his standards.Today, Ferragamo shoes are sold worldwide and have the reputation of being among the most comfortable of women's footwear.

High-heeled shoes of three or more inches continued to be popular until World War Two—when function and material shortages determined styles—and included wedge platform styles with cork arch supports, reminiscent of those worn by the actors in ancient Greece.At the same time, many shoe manufacturers specialized in flats and advertised that high-heeled shoes caused illnesses from headaches to nausea to constipation.They had the right idea but the wrong complaints.

As far as I am concerned, the big trouble in this century began in the 1950s with the advent of the stiletto heel. The style had its birth in Italy and France and eventually made its disastrous way to North America. Since then we have had all types of footwear, with all sorts of heels, toe-boxes, and shapes. As I have said throughout this book, these shoes are responsible for exacerbating or even causing a multitude of sins. Although I will have much to say about footwear in general, I devote much of the remainder of this chapter to the pros and cons of various types of athletic shoes, because they have become the first choice in footwear for so many people today.

## Last Is First

Regardless of the type of footwear under discussion, analysis must begin with the last, the form from which shoes are made. That form is the shape of a human foot. Today, with the mass production of shoes, lasts are designed to provide footwear for the "average" man and woman. Unfortunately, not all of us are average. Also, shoe manufacturers often have trouble determining just what is average. This is particularly true in the case of fashion footwear. Can it be that our wide forefeet are just an optical illusion, and that our toes really can fit into those low, tiny toe-boxes? Moreover, at least one-fifth of all women have a wide forefoot and a narrow heel. Yet try to find a sensible, fashionable pair of shoes in all sizes for that 20 per cent. It's not easy. What is required is a combination-last shoe, which incorporates a wider forefoot with a narrower heel. It would be simple enough to do, but at an increase in production costs for a smaller market. Shoe manufacturers are in the business to make a healthy profit. Unless they are in the athletic or specialty shoe business, fashion comes first and healthy feet come second. Which is maybe why more people are switching to comfortable, sensible athletic or walking shoes for regular wear.

## Too Many Shoes Foil the Browser

Have you walked into a sporting goods or athletic shoe store recently and been overwhelmed by the different types of footwear on the shelves? Well, you're not alone. There are now shoes for different types of running (long-distance, cross-country, sprinting) and tennis shoes for all the various surfaces from grass to clay to artificial. There are shoes for different track-and-field events, for high- and low-impact aerobics, baseball, football, basketball, soccer, and a host of other indoor and outdoor activities. And most of them also have different tread designs for different types of surfaces.To further confuse the prospective buyer, many athletic shoe manufacturers are now making walking shoes for those who want the benefits of running shoes but with a little style. Since, as I have already noted, about 90 per cent of today's purchasers of athletic shoes want them for casual wear, there is an obvious market for the walking variety.

## Running Shoes

Although it was as far back as 1909 when the first real pair of running shoes was produced, it is only in the past few years that the shoes have been designed specifically for certain activities and foot problems. When the running craze took off in the early 1970s, two German footwear manufacturers—Adidas and Puma—were the only major players on the scene to cash in immediately on the demand for running shoes. Today there are well over thirty major athletic shoe manufacturers in the world, and the top three are now grossing over $1 billion in sales each year.These companies have developed tremendous resources to research, manufacture, and market the ultimate in athletic footwear. Their space-age laboratories have enabled them to produce soft, lightweight, comfortable shoes with excellent shock-absorption to suit every need (see Diagram 13). Many of the companies in the United States have research centers to determine average foot abnormalities so that their shoes can help correct those problems.

These companies have learned from the mistake of trying to alter the angle of the foot in the shoe, or repositioning the foot in the shoe. The trick is to keep the foot in the "neutral" position, to help prevent abnormal pronation. (A neutral position does not tilt the foot in any way to promote abnormal pronation or supination.) They also understand that good stability in the shoe will help prevent over-pronation, and many of them place stabilizing bars in their shoes—for example, on the inside part of the heel where over-pronation often occurs.

When Brooks came out with their Chariot line, they promoted the dual-density feature of the shoes. The rubber on the big toe side of these shoes is muchstiffer than on the baby toe side. The idea is to provide the added stability on the big toe side of the foot when the forefoot is in contact with the ground, while providing flexibility on the baby toe side. Brooks also came out in the mid-1980s with the "kinetic wedge" under the big toe joint. Their reasoning was that the soft wedge would enable that part of the foot to sink lower down and thereby help prevent some pronation. The kinetic wedge works well for many people, but as with any athletic shoe, it must be appropriate for your type of foot to be successful.

Another concern for athletic shoe manufacturers, besides preventing over-pronation, is shock absorption. There is

Diagram 13
## The Anatomy of a Running Shoe

Upper gives stability,
flexibility and breathability

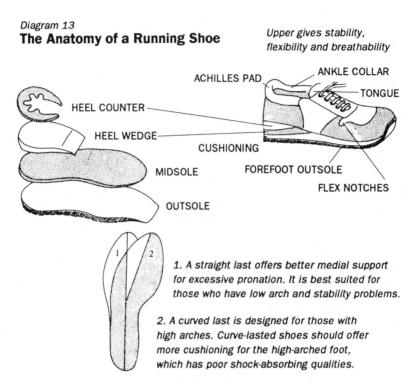

ACHILLES PAD

ANKLE COLLAR

TONGUE

HEEL COUNTER

HEEL WEDGE

CUSHIONING

MIDSOLE

FOREFOOT OUTSOLE

FLEX NOTCHES

OUTSOLE

1. A straight last offers better medial support
for excessive pronation. It is best suited for
those who have low arch and stability problems.

2. A curved last is designed for those with
high arches. Curve-lasted shoes should offer
more cushioning for the high-arched foot,
which has poor shock-absorbing qualities.

a need to cushion the lower part of the body from the constant jarring of running and walking. The less stress on the bones and joints, the less likelihood of wear and tear and overuse syndromes. To give you that feeling of walking on air, Nike produced the Air line of athletic footwear, which have air pockets at the bottom from the rearfoot to the midfoot. Not to be outdone, Tiger came out with the Tiger Gels, which uses a gel instead of air in the pockets, and Brooks introduced their HydroFlow line with water replacing the air or gel. Some people may dismiss all these concepts as gimmicky, although there are those who claim that their Nike Airs or similar shoes are the most comfortable they have ever worn. Moreover, there is no doubt that these shoes provide good flexibility and stability, as well as excellent shock absorption.

When it comes to stability, many young, active individuals swear by their Reebok "pumps", high-top shoes with an air bladder that can be pumped up or released to mold perfectly to the shape of the foot. These shoes do provide excellent ankle support, but I suspect the same molding feature can be achieved in most athletic shoes that have sophisticated lacing systems, which allow the fit to be as tight or as loose as desired.

All these shoes have their merits. Often the selection boils down to which last fits your foot best, since most of the shoes provide good shock absorption, flexibility, and stability. One thing to keep in mind is that heavier, taller people will naturally require more shock absorption and stability in their shoes than smaller persons. Therefore, they should ascertain (perhaps with the help of a knowledgeable salesperson) which shoes are best suited to their frame. I would strongly recommend that you try on as many pairs of shoes as possible (on both feet) to ensure that all your needs are met.

### Cross-training Shoes

Cross-trainers are meant for those who like to dabble in various types of exercises but who don't want to spend a fortune for shoes designed specifically for each one of their activities. Cross-trainers are quite suitable for persons who run no more than 30 miles (50 km) a week, play fewer than three hours of tennis a day, and do some bicycle riding and/or aerobics. These shoes are built to provide adequate stability, shock absorption, and flexibility for all those activities. Considering that only one in ten athletic shoe buyers today is a serious athlete, it is understandable that cross-trainers have captured a large share of the market. They may be the closest thing today to the PF Flyers my peers and I wore when we were growing up.

The major difference between cross-trainers and running shoes is that the latter have more built-in stability and rearfoot shock absorption, which are required for more serious running. Cross-trainers may be slightly more flexible to allow for a wider range of foot motions required in disparate activities. They may also have more shock absorption in the forefoot to provide cushioning for activities such as aerobics and racquet sports that place greater stress on the front part of the foot. For the individual who wants to buy a pair of athletic shoes to walk in, I would make my choice between the two types based on comfort and style. I would choose either a running shoe or cross-trainer over a walking shoe. The latter is actually a cross between an oxford and a running shoe, and as such it does not have the same amount of stability and support as an athletic shoe. Also, it is usually much more expensive. However, I would certainly recommend a walking shoe over fashion footwear for everyday use.

### Aerobic Shoes

Are aerobic shoes really better for this exercise than running shoes? Recent studies in the United States indicate that they aren't, an argument I have been championing for years.

Last summer I treated a patient for a sprained ankle, incurred while she was doing high-impact aerobics. Her instructor blamed her accident on her running shoes. This is nonsense, because there is more support in the ankle in running shoes than in aerobic shoes. Had she been wearing aerobic shoes she would probably have suffered greater rather than less damage to her ankle when she tripped.

Aerobic shoes do provide better control in the forefoot than running shoes do. They are heavier and have thicker rubber in the sole, as well as more padding under the forefoot. However, they do not have quite the same side-to-side stability of running shoes, which may account for the ankle sprains that can occur during some aerobic exercise routines. One option for those who want to wear aerobic shoes is the Avia high-top, which does provide additional ankle support. The main advantage of aerobic shoes is their treads, which differ from those of running shoes and have a better grip for hardwood floors. (Incidentally, you may marvel at all the tread variations you see on the different athletic shoes. Some of them may grip different surfaces better than others. On the whole, however, the tread on the shoe is far less important than the three major considerations—shock absorption, flexibility, and stability.) For low-impact aerobics, a comfortable pair of cross-trainers would be quite suitable. Since there is significantly less stress on the foot and lower leg than in high-impact aerobics, the type of athletic footwear is less important.

### Racquet-Sport Shoes
Racquet sports require a lot of lateral motion, so shoes for these sports must have excellent stability to keep the feet as "neutral" as possible as they slide from side to side and often come to a jarring stop, which places enormous stress on the outside part of the feet. Typical squash court

shoes, for example, will have an extra-rigid layer of material around the heel and forefoot to provide that added stability. Tennis players are subjected to added stress on their sesamoids when they serve, so they should wear shoes that provide extra protection for that part of the foot.All other types of athletic footwear are designed specifically for certain activities.Generally, though, when you are shopping for a good pair of athletic shoes, you need not waste your time and energies on the esoteric models.Stick to the cross-trainers and running shoes and you will not go wrong.

### Trends

Athletic footwear will undoubtedly continue to improve as manufacturers continue to pump millions of dollars into research to stay ahead of the competition.However, I suspect that the selection of specialized athletic shoes will diminish in the next few years as the quality of cross-trainers improves.Moreover, even the most specialized stores will not be able to handle so much esoteric merchandise profitably.I also anticipate fewer shoes designed specifically for marathon running and high-impact aerobics, since both activities are on the decline.

### Fashion Statements

Throughout this book I have discussed fashion shoes and the harm they can do. Fortunately, I sense a trend towards footwear that does not cause or exacerbate a foot abnormality.We should be thankful that youngsters today are into high-top athletic shoes rather than something like negative-heel shoes. I have also noticed over the past few years that many of the major brands of women's footwear include sensibly designed shoes with lower heels and larger toe-boxes.There is even a wider variety of these better-fitting shoes available for those with non-average feet. But we must remember that the number-one priority of the fashion shoe is to make a fashion statement, so we cannot yet expect a woman's dress shoe to provide adequate stability, flexibility, and shock absorption for constant wear.

When it comes to footwear, men remain better off than women. The styles rarely change significantly; heel heights are consistently in the optimum one-inch area; comfort is perhaps more of a selling feature than with women's shoes; and most stores offer a wide range of sizes and widths from which to choose. My primary suggestion for men is that, if they are wearing orthotics, laced shoes will accommodate the inserts much more easily than loafers.

### Kiddy Corner

A controversy continues to rage in pediatric circles about whether a child is better off in high-top oxfords or in running shoes. Many orthopods and podiatrists favor the oxfords, because they offer more stability. Others, like myself, believe that running shoes provide more than adequate stability and offer much greater flexibility and comfort for the growing foot.I suppose the high-top basketball shoes that Michael Jordan, et al., promote may provide the best of both worlds for most children. My three kids are growing up on running shoes, because I feel that flexibility is the most important consideration in children's footwear. And they have not developed any foot problems.

There is no need for infants to wear shoes until they are

walking constantly. Socks are fine, as long as they are not too tight and are made of natural fibers—cotton or wool—which absorb perspiration. If you are afraid that your baby's feet are cold without shoes, you are worrying needlessly. In cold weather, there are better ways to keep feet warm than with constricting shoes.

### Orthotics

Custom-made leather devices were inserted in shoes for reasons of comfort as far back as the fifteenth century. In the early 1900s in Europe, custom-designed arch supports became popular and even today are commonly sold on the Continent in ordinary shoe stores. They are manufactured to specific sizes and many feature additional frills such as cork or added leather to increase comfort.

After World War Two, laboratories in the United States began researching and custom-making leather orthotics. These inserts were prescribed by podiatrists and other medical specialists who would take an impression of the patient's feet and send it to the laboratory. Most of the impressions were made in a plaster cast, and subsequently in foam, a procedure that is still the norm today.

The laboratories advanced in the early 1970s to the point where they were effectively replacing leather with harder, more rigid materials, usually different types of plastic. These newer orthotics were thinner, took up less space in the shoe, and provided excellent correction for foot abnormalities. Then, as the running craze mushroomed throughout North America, the need arose for softer orthotics. So the laboratories developed softer plastics, which provided increased flexibility and shock absorption but maintained corrective properties. Until recently

European manufacturers stuck with leather custom-designed (rather than custom-made) inserts. Custom-designed inserts are mass-produced for specific types of feet and footwear. Custom-made inserts are the equivalent of made-to-measure clothing; they are based on the requirements of one person. In North America custom-designed inserts are only now being marketed as an alternative to prescribed orthotics, while in Europe laboratories have begun to custom-make orthotics. I remain convinced that for people with definite foot problems, a custom-made orthotic will provide far superior abnormality correction than the custom-designed models.

There are now more than two hundred compounds being used for different types of orthotics. I believe that in the not too distant future new materials, or a combination of existing ones, will provide the ultimate in correction, shock absorption, flexibility, and durability. At present I prefer custom-made graphite orthotics. Graphite is very flexible, quite thin, and fits most shoes much better than other materials. The bulkier orthotics of the past did perhaps provide somewhat better foot control, but people did not wear them regularly, because they either were too uncomfortable or did not fit all their shoes. I would rather have them worn continuously and give 80 per cent of the control all of the time than worn 30 per cent of the time with 100 per cent control. The "fashion" orthotics available today in graphite will fit almost all women's shoes comfortably, including high-heels.

However, graphite tends to crack more easily than other materials, though it holds the foot stable in the "neutral" position, provides flexibility, adequate shock absorption, and (if it doesn't crack) is usually more durable than other materials, which may wear well for only a few months before breaking down.When the material breaks down the insert obviously loses its abilities to function adequately.

One of my patients has been wearing orthotics for about six years. Her first pair lasted for over one year, then began to break down. She knew that something was wrong with them because her calluses returned and her feet began to hurt again. After that the orthotics had to be rebuilt or replaced almost every six months, for she was on her feet a good deal of the time and was very uncomfortable without them. A year ago I prescribed a new pair of graphite orthotics and they have stood up much better than her old ones.

It is essential to follow a proper regimen when breaking in a new pair of orthotics. They must be worn for only a couple of hours on the first day. Then the time is gradually increased until they can be left in the shoes all day. It takes a while for your body to become accustomed to walking differently, and if you wear the inserts too long at the beginning you will probably develop aches and pains throughout your lower extremities.Should that happen you may erroneously believe that the orthotics are bad for you and discontinue wearing them.That would be a serious mistake.

In the past few years non-medical "experts" have begun dispensing orthotics.The inserts are even occasionally advertised by mail-order operations in magazines and newspapers.Would you allow yourself to be fitted for contact lenses by someone without university training, or purchase them sight unseen (pardon the pun) through the mail? I hope the answer is a resounding "no!" As with your eyesight, there are no bargains or "snake oil" remedies when proper foot care is involved. In some of the states in the U.S. non-professionals are prohibited from dispensing orthotics. Unfortunately, such is not the case anywhere in Canada.

If you are having foot problems and believe that you may require custom-made orthotics, see a licensed podiatrist first for an evaluation. You may be able to get cheaper inserts elsewhere, but your feet deserve the best, not an inadequate bargain. If you need other medical care, the podiatrist will not hesitate to refer you to the proper specialist.

# 9

# POPPING THE QUESTIONS

THERE ARE TWO SECTIONS OF QUESTIONS AND answers in this chapter.The first section focuses on systemic diseases that can have an adverse effect on lower extremities. The second section answers some of the most common questions regarding foot care.

Systemic diseases can adversely affect your lower extremities. You have already been given a peek at some of the potential problem areas when I discussed geriatric concerns in detail in Chapter Six. I should point out that some of my patients have a combination of systemic disorders and biomechanical problems.Unfortunately, the biomechanical faults are often forgotten or overlooked while the disease processes are being aggressively treated.

## SYSTEMS ANALYSIS

**Q.** I have psoriatic arthritis. Can this cause pain on the bottom of my foot?

**A.** The answer to your question is no.I recently had a patient who suffered simultaneously from psoriatic arthritis and plantar fasciitis.Psoriatic arthritis is a disease that affects a small number of people who have psoriasis and is usually manifested by mild to severe outbreaks in various joints. However, it can attack the entire body and often mimics rheumatoid arthritis, and should be treated by a rheumatologist.

Diane was diagnosed as having psoriatic arthritis two years ago.She was experiencing pain, stiffness, and swelling of her toe joints. Her doctor gave her an anti-inflammatory drug, which totally relieved the symptoms, and she resumed her normal lifestyle, which included aerobics and daily long walks. In December 1989 she was walking barefoot on a Caribbean beach when her feet began to hurt.The pain gradually worsened over the next two weeks, her ankle and toe joints swelled, and she began having great difficulty walking. Her doctors switched her medication, and she went to physiotherapy three times a week for three months.But all the ice and ultrasound could not completely relieve her symptoms. A customer in a shoe store told Diane about her podiatrist, and she decided to make an appointment to see me.

It was quite obvious to me that Diane was suffering from plantar fasciitis (which had been overlooked) as well as psoriatic arthritis.I prescribed orthotics for her and saw her regularly last spring and summer to ensure that the orthotics were working. Although she still has some arthritic pain, for which she takes medication, her plantar fasciitis has disappeared. Unfortunately, Diane suffered needlessly for months because it was thought that all her problems were being caused by psoriatic arthritis.

**Q.** I recently saw a commercial on television for a product that treated athlete's foot. The advertisement claimed that I could get a secondary yeast infection if I did not use the proper medication (theirs, I assume).  Is that true?

**A.** Strictly speaking, yeast is a type of fungus. However, yeast and the fungus that causes athlete's foot are different. And it is true that if you have athlete's foot you can develop a secondary yeast infection.To complicate matters, you could develop a bacterial infection as well. So any medication you apply to the affected area ought to be anti-bacterial as well as anti-fungal. As far as anti-fungal medications are concerned, most of them will take care of both yeast and athlete's foot infections.Your pharmacist ought to be able to help you find the right product.If the infection persists you will require the help of a medical professional and, perhaps, stronger medication that can be dispensed only with a prescription.

**Q.** Why is it that diabetics are so prone to foot infections, which can become gangrenous?

**A.** Two of the unfortunate side effects of diabetes may be the early onset of atherosclerosis, a buildup of plaque in the arteries, and arteriosclerosis, a hardening of the arteries.These conditions result in diminished blood circulation, and are worst in parts of the body farthest from the heart—particularly the feet. When an area has been injured or infected it requires a sufficient amount of fresh blood carrying oxygen, white blood cells that attack the bacteria, and healing nutrients in order to recover.If an infection cannot be killed it will most likely spread or cause serious damage to the part of the body it has attacked. Gangrene occurs when body tissue dies, which can be a result of, for example, a massive infection or severe frostbite.When diabetics develop a foot infection they must seek immediate medical attention if they suspect that they might also be suffering from poor circulation.

Of course diabetics will not automatically develop gangrene if they get an infected toe.Those who take good care of themselves may well avoid atherosclerosis.But even the lucky ones must take the proper precautions to minimize the risk of a foot infection.If I were diabetic I would examine my feet regularly to ensure that I was not developing an infection.I would avoid "bathroom" surgery to remove such things as corns and ingrown nails, because one tiny slip of the knife or scissors could lead to a bacterial infection. I would also stay far away from any acid-based medications or pads to treat corns or calluses. Acids can cause skin lesions that can quickly become infected.

A typical example of how diabetes can turn a biomechanical foot problem into a serious health problem is a sixty-two-year-old patient of mine. Harry was diagnosed as a borderline diabetic in 1967 and was treated with oral medications.A few years later he suffered a hairline fracture of a metatarsal bone, which was followed by severe callusing of the ball of his left foot under the site of the fracture. The area became increasingly painful and in 1983 his personal physician referred him to a podiatrist, who diagnosed his condition as a "diabetic ulcer." He periodically had the callus trimmed and was provided with a pad with a cotton loop to protect the inflamed area. In 1987 the chafing of the loop caused a lesion in the skin, which then became severely infected.Because of this man's diabetes he was hospitalized for two weeks and kept on intravenous antibiotics. He was told at the hospital that the pad and loop no longer sufficed and that he required alternative treatment for his foot problems.

It was after Harry's release from hospital that I first treated him. I diagnosed his condition as one of dropped metatarsal heads and advised him that he would require on-going care because further ulceration of the ball of the foot was possible. Shortly thereafter he developed an inflamed callus under the fourth metatarsal head and was immediately examined by an orthopedic surgeon, who specializes in foot surgery, and an endocrinologist who specialized in diabetes.We jointly decided that surgery be performed immediately to raise the fourth metatarsal head, and it was completed successfully. However, it took three further operations to correct similar problems with the first and second metatarsal heads. Fortunately, the situation finally seems to have stabilized and Harry has not experienced any difficulties recently. The chances of a recurrence of the ulcerated calluses will depend on his biomechanics, and for that reason he now wears orthotics all the time. He also applies cream daily to the ball of his foot to keep the skin from cracking. Finally, I examine his feet regularly to ensure that no other potentially dangerous infection materializes.

**Q.** I have been told that I suffer from intermittent claudication, which makes walking quite difficult for me. What can I do to overcome this problem?

**A.** Claudication is caused by poor circulation.Blood flow to the lower legs, particularly to the calf muscles, is insufficient for a variety of reasons. When the calf muscles fail to receive a sufficient amount of blood they cry out for oxygen.You get the message clearly in the form of loud cramping pain, which will normally occur five to ten minutes after you have begun walking.At that point you will have to sit down for a few minutes until the pain subsides.Many people with the disorder find that their relief is enhanced by rubbing the painful area.Then you can get up again and walk pain-free until the cramps hit once more—if they do return.The resting routine is then repeated and the pain subsides, which is why the condition is called intermittent claudication.

The first thing a person ought to do when this disorder is suspected is have a complete physical examination to determine the origin and seriousness of the circulation problem, if, indeed, circulatory disease is the culprit, which is not always the case. Once the systemic condition has been diagnosed and treatment has begun, the person should undertake a supervised exercise program, which will eventually allow him or her to walk pain-free for long periods.

**Q.** I froze my toes when I was a youngster, and they have remained ultra-sensitive to cold. Since I love to ski, I would like to know how I can best prevent a recurrence of the pain every time I hit the slopes.

**A.** When a person suffers frostbite—as you have apparently done—some of the tiny blood vessels at the end of the toes are permanently damaged. This means that blood circulation to the tips of the toes is diminished. In cold weather vasoconstriction (narrowing) of the blood vessels occurs naturally, which further reduces blood flow to the feet. So when you are out on the slopes your toes are not receiving sufficient blood, and, after a while, they scream bloody murder at you to warn you that they are about to freeze again.

There are two ways to avoid the agony of freezing toes. First, wear properly insulated ski boots and an extra pair of heavy socks. Secondly, warm and rest your feet indoors every couple of hours. On very cold days it would be wise not to stay out on the slopes for too long. A little common sense can save you a mountain of pain.

**Q.** My great-uncle always suffered from gout. He had a large red spot on the big toe side of his foot. Is that indicative of a bunion? If so, do all people with gout get bunions?

**A.** Gout is an excess of uric acid in the blood. Uric acid crystals tend to settle in parts of the body farthest from the center of the circulatory system—the heart—and have a real affinity for the big toe joint. These crystals create friction in the joint, much as sand does when it gets into a ball-bearing joint in a piece of machinery. The results of this friction in the big toe joint are acute inflammation and swelling, which cause the redness in the area and mimic the symptoms of a bunion. Gout is a systemic disorder and is treated by medication and diet to lower the uric acid level in the blood. It does not cause bunions.

**Q.** I am a pensioner with swollen ankles. I went to the doctor to get some water pills, but he wouldn't prescribe them. Instead he told me to wear support hose. Why?

**A.** As people age, it is natural for their circulatory systems to function less efficiently than when they were young.Your veins and valves may have weakened sufficiently to affect the flow of blood from your feet back to your heart. By the end of the day, and if you have been on your feet quite a bit, the fluid that cannot get back to the heart will build up in your lower extremities. Blame the forces of gravity, not your doctor, for your swollen ankles, where much of this fluid has settled. Support hose restrict the amount of room in your lower legs and feet for retaining this fluid.They also help the muscles contract, which assists your veins in their attempt to pump the blood back to the heart. Water pills may not be the answer to your problems, particularly if you are not retaining water to excess. Also, this type of medication may not be without some side effects.

If you have consistently swollen ankles, you should be examined by your physician to determine the exact cause of your condition. There are a number of reasons why your ankles may be swelling, other than water retention.

**Q.** I had bypass surgery about eighteen months ago, and my ankles keep swelling up. According to my family physician, this is due to the "harvesting" of veins in my feet for use in the operation. Can you explain this relationship between my surgery and my swollen ankles?

**A.** Many people who have had bypass surgery had veins from their legs used to replace damaged or clogged coronary arteries. The procedure is similar to having varicose veins stripped. As a result, other veins in the legs must take up the slack, and they are not always capable of functioning as well as the veins "harvested" for the bypass operation. Therefore, 'he return flow of blood from your feet to your heart is not as efficient as it once was, and fluid builds up in your ankles.

**Q.** I have been a smoker all my adult life.I now have circulatory problems in my feet. My doctor says that my three-pack-a-day habit for forty-five years is the cause of my discomfort.What does smoking have to do with my bum feet?

**A.** Smoking is widely implicated in arteriosclerosis (hardening of the arteries) and atherosclerosis (a buildup of plaque in the arteries). As with other circulatory diseases, the symptoms first appear in an area farthest from the heart, namely, the feet. What you have is a systemic disorder caused by damage to the blood vessels in your lower extremities, including your feet. Smoking affects the entire body, not just the lungs and heart. Repair is not easy, or even possible, once the damage has been done to the blood vessels. Therefore, the best way to prevent this problem is not to smoke!

**Q.** I have been a heavy drinker for the last twenty years. I am now fifty-two years old, and I have had a burning sensation in my feet for the past few months.My family doctor told me I have alcoholic neuropathy of the feet. What is it, and can it be cured?

**A.** One of the unpleasant side effects of alcoholism is neuritis, an inflammation of the nerves, which is common in the lower legs and feet of long-time abusers of alcohol. This condition is not well understood, but is thought to be similar to diabetic neuropathy, in which diabetics tend to convert glucose into sorbitol, a carbohydrate that the body is unable to break down. Sorbitol seems to have an affinity for nerve endings and causes inflammation, which in turn creates the burning sensation.As for alcoholic neuropathy, an ounce of prevention is worth the proverbial pound of cure. In fact, there is no cure at this time.

**Q.** I am a seventy-three-year-old lady who has developed dark brown spots just above both ankle bones. A dermatologist told me that my problem was circulatory. What do these spots have to do with my circulation?

**A.** This condition is known as stasis dermatitis.It is caused by a buildup of fluid or poor arterial function in the lower extremities. As a result insufficient oxygen is reaching cells of the skin—in your case just above the ankle bones.The skin discolors because of this oxygen insufficiency. This may, in fact, be the first indication of a circulatory disorder. Little can be done to get rid of the brown spots. However, the early detection of a circulatory condition can prevent the onset of more severe problems. The appearance of such spots should spur you into seeing your doctor for a complete physical examination.

**Q.** My doctor told me that the circulation in my lower legs is bad and that I should walk as much as possible. Shouldn't I be doing just the opposite?

**A.** You probably do have poor circulation. Your doctor has determined that you would benefit from the increased exercise to force "collateral circulation." The idea is to force auxiliary vessels in your lower extremities to work so that they will expand to allow for greater blood flow. If a blood vessel is made to work harder it will eventually expand and take up the slack caused by other dysfunctional vessels in the area. Intermittent claudication is one condition that often benefits from such a regimen. As with all other circulatory problems, your doctor will be able to advise the course of action to take.

**Q.** I read that osteoarthritis may actually be caused by a collagen disorder, and is, therefore, a disease, not a wear-and-tear problem. Is this true?

**A.** As I was writing this book a report appeared that researchers had isolated a gene that was somehow linked to osteoarthritis. This defective gene seems to cause an early breakdown of collagen, a fibrous protein found in cartilage. The researchers are quite excited by their findings. I will wait until the results of further research are published before making up my mind. Even if a disease link to osteoarthritis is proved, it will take a lengthy period of genetic engineering research to develop a treatment process to eliminate or reverse the effects of this gene.

I would speculate that some people may indeed be more susceptible to a more rapid wear-and-tear process in certain joints.This may be due to some genetic defect and could be compared with that of a tire that is manufactured with a slight flaw.That defect will eventually cause the tire to wear out more quickly than normal.However, I still believe that osteoarthritis is primarily a wear-and-tear disorder.By the time this book is published, additional research may have come to light to refute either my beliefs or those of the researchers to which you referred.

**Q.** I am constantly getting cramps on the bottoms of my feet and in my calves. Sometimes I wake up in the middle of the night in agony from the cramping. What is causing these cramps, and I how can I avoid them?

**A.** This is a difficult question to answer. Cramping may be caused by muscle tightness, or overuse (a buildup of lactic acid in the muscle), and activated by over-stretching while you are sleeping. This type of cramping was once thought to be due to insufficient calcium in the body, but this theory has few followers today. Quinine has been used to counter the problem for many years, with a modicum of success. Occasionally, there may be a circulatory or diabetes component involved; but I would not be too concerned, even if I knew I already suffered from either disorder. Once again, I would advise that a visit to the doctor is in order here to determine the cause of the problem.

**Q.** I have multiple sclerosis and am suffering from plantar fasciitis. Is this a result of M.S.? Should I be treated by my neurologist or a podiatrist for the foot problem?

**A.** It is not unusual for a person with multiple sclerosis (M.S.) to get plantar fasciitis. This is because people with M.S. tend to develop an abnormal gait, because of motor nerve damage that affects their lower extremities, causing the plantar fasciae to twist and over-stretch. Treatment for plantar fasciitis involves rest, ice, orthotics, ultrasound, and anti-inflammatory medication if required. It would be wise to have the podiatrist co-ordinate treatment with the neurologist to ensure the best possible course of action and to avoid inappropriate medications.

I have one patient, Joan, who is a fairly typical example of how M.S. can affect the lower extremities. She was diagnosed with the disease in 1967, when she was thirty-three. At the time she was pregnant, and had always led a very active life—boating, camping, alpine skiing. In 1972 she was hospitalized with a severe bladder infection and also lost her sight for a while. Moreover, she lost much of her motor function in her right leg and foot. She was gradually able to walk with a brace on her right leg and with the help of a cane. By 1983 the toes on her feet had curled, causing the tips of her toes to become skinned whenever she wore shoes. An orthopedic surgeon performed a tendon transplant procedure to straighten out the toes. For six weeks she hobbled about in walking casts, with two canes, and with pins in her toes. Unfortunately, she still had curled and painful toes on her left foot, and she underwent further surgery to fuse three of the toes.

The pain in Joan's left foot steadily increased. "At times my left foot could have a spasm, which extended up my leg and made my knee buckle, resulting in a fall." Her right foot was not much better, and it turned sideways. Her legs were becoming misshapen and swollen, and the pain was endless, often disturbing her sleep.

Joan's misery continued throughout the mid-1980s, despite the intervention of orthopedic and neuro-surgeons and physical therapists. One therapist suggested that she wear shoes one size larger. Joan did so, and began tripping and falling because the shoes did not fit properly. In May 1990 she was seen by a doctor at a hospital foot clinic. She was advised to wear inserts in her athletic shoes. She thought it was a ridiculous suggestion, particularly since she could not wear such footwear with "a black dinner dress." She then went to an acupuncture pain clinic where she experienced some relief from her pain and swelling. The doctor there referred her to me. At this point she had so much pain when she walked that she thought M.S. "was going to win."

I agreed that Joan required inserts for her shoes, and ordered custom-made orthotics for her. Once she began wearing the orthotics, the pain and swelling in her legs and feet decreased substantially. The shape of her legs has returned to normal. "I'm no longer afraid to walk," she told me on her last visit to my office. "It's hard to believe that a short time ago I felt it wouldn't be the M.S. that would put me in a wheel chair, but my feet!" The orthotics have sufficiently corrected the biomechanics in her feet so that she is now able to walk again.

**Q.** I have been told that my foot problems are caused by Marfan syndrome, a disease I apparently inherited. Can you explain the relationship between this disorder and bad feet?

**A.** I am well acquainted with Marfan syndrome. I have had a patient since 1980 who has suffered greatly from this disorder.

Marfan syndrome is an inherited disorder that affects the body's connective tissue. It is characterized by excessive height and unusually long and slender fingers and toes, as well as long arms and legs. It can also cause severe heart and eye defects. It affects the feet and legs because the ligaments, muscles, and tendons become too weak to support weight properly. I can illustrate by reciting the case history of my patient.

Jill is now forty-nine years old. Her shoe size is 13 AAAA! She has high, weak arches and terrible biomechanics. In 1980 she was referred to me by her family physician, who believed that her "flat feet" were throwing her knees, hips, and spine out of alignment, which would inevitably create arthritic problems as she got older. I prescribed orthotics for her and the results were very positive.

In 1988 the connective tissue in her aorta became so weak that most of the artery had to be replaced with a plastic blood vessel. She also required the replacement of the renal and celiac arteries. During the complicated operation a nerve was damaged and she was left partially paralyzed from the hips down. Three months of intensive physiotherapy enabled her to "stand and shuffle short distances, with the aid of two canes." However, her feet were extremely painful because she was literally walking on her ankles. It turned out that she had suffered severe tendon damage in her feet when she was first trying to walk again.

Jill was not willing to live with the problem until her legs got stronger and her balance improved, as she was told she must at the rehabilitation hospital, so, once she was released she returned to see me. It took many visits and several types of orthotics, but we finally found one insert that was strong enough to support her weight but soft and pliable enough not to hurt her feet. Jill can now work longer and harder at her physiotherapy program and she can walk farther even though she is still partially paralyzed down the back and inside of both legs.

Jill is not quite typical of most Marfan syndrome sufferers because of the complications she suffered as a result of her surgery. However, she is typical of the people who can function and walk fairly pain-free even though they have been struck by a potentially debilitating illness.

**Q.** My family doctor told me that I had osteoarthritis in my big toe. A while ago I was diagnosed by a rheumatologist as having rheumatoid arthritis in my right knee. Can I get both types of arthritis at the same time?

**A.** Yes. Rheumatoid arthritis normally attacks the larger joints in the body—the shoulders, the hips, the knees. Osteoarthritis, a wear-and-tear disorder, affects large and small joints alike. It is not unusual to have rheumatoid arthritis in one knee and osteoarthritis in one toe. Blood tests can identify the presence of rheumatoid arthritis. Osteoarthritis can be detected by x-rays and bone-scanning devices. The diagnostic tests can be verified when the patients are examined by doctors who are well versed in arthritic disorders.

**Q.** I have had plantar warts for what seems like an eternity. I have had them burned out with acid twice, surgically removed once, and zapped with a laser once. But they keep returning! Will I be plagued by them for life?

**A.** Plantar warts are caused by the papilloma virus, which somehow gets under your skin on the bottom of your foot. The thing to remember is that the body's defense systems will eventually hunt down and kill the virus, at which time the wart will disappear. Unfortunately, it sometimes takes a few years for your virus fighters to kill the papilloma virus. Sometimes plantar warts can last for many years even if treated.

It is important to ensure that any treatment does not leave scar tissue on the bottom of the foot. A scarred weight-bearing part of the foot can be a painful place indeed, and will probably cause the sufferer to alter his gait in order to avoid the agony. Once he begins to walk abnormally he will develop a biomechanical problem, which will only make his feet even sorer and could even affect his legs, knees, hips, and lower back. There are many "snake oil" remedies for plantar warts, all of them less damaging than the application of strong acids, the laser beam, or the knife. Many people seem to have actually succeeded in getting rid of their plantar warts with a regular application of cod liver oil for about five weeks.

If you have unsuccessfully tried all sorts of remedies and approaches in your quest to eliminate forever your plantar warts, you should try a mild acid solution as prescribed by your dermatologist or podiatrist. I would be reluctant to take stronger action because of the possibility of producing significant permanent scarring. I also counsel my patients to live with the warts if they are not causing any pain, until they go away naturally.Some minor discomfort could be alleviated by wearing a soft pad under the infected area.

One word of advice—and this applies to all types of foot problems whether they be caused by systemic disorders or biomechanical abnormalities. Have your foot examined by a specialist to ensure that what you think is a plantar wart really is a plantar wart.It is not that difficult to misdiagnose a wart as a callus, and vice versa. If you have been unsuccessful in getting rid of your plantar warts using home remedies, it may be because you actually have a callus, which will consistently return as long as the biomechanical fault causing it is not eliminated.

## Common Questions on Foot Care

**Q.** I hurt my ankle two months ago.Though it seems to have healed, I still get a sharp pain at least once a day while I am walking. Why?

**A.** Whenever you sprain your ankle, it is quite common for at least one of the three major ankle ligaments to become over-stretched and inflamed.Inflammation leads to swelling in the area, which is how the body limits motion in a joint to prevent it from becoming further damaged. Most people believe that the sprain has healed when the swelling disappears.It ain't necessarily so!

If the sprain is moderate to severe, the site of the injury must be strengthened before it will return to normal. Just walking will not sufficiently strengthen the ankle joint.This is because the affected ligament or ligaments have been damaged or weakened by the injury.

The first step in treating an injured ankle is the old standby, r.i.c.e.—rest, ice, compression, elevation. Once the pain and swelling have subsided, the next step is to begin strengthening the over-stretched ligaments with the proper physiotherapy program.But there is another reason for aggressively treating an ankle sprain—jangled nerves. Some nerves transmit pain signals; others (motor nerves) send and receive messages from the brain that enable us to move.When you sprain your ankle you damage motor (proprioceptor) nerves in the area.The proprioceptor nerves there normally feed to the brain accurate information about what part of your foot is in contact with the ground at a given moment.When these nerves are damaged they are no longer able to send a clear, accurate signal to the brain, which obviously cannot then react properly to provide information to enable you to walk normally. As a result you may stumble and resprain your ankle. Physiotherapy to repair the proprioceptors must begin as soon as possible after the injury and should be part of a comprehensive therapy program to rebuild and strengthen the ankle joint.

**Q.** A friend recently underwent electromagnetic therapy for a sore foot. How does it work? Can it cure my arthritic knee?

**A.** The therapeutic benefits of electromagnetic forces have been extensively studied in the past twenty years, particularly in Europe. Initial research was aimed at treating bone fractures that would not heal (non-union). A negative-charged plate was placed on one piece of the fractured bone and a positive plate on the other piece of the bone.Electromagnetic waves were then applied to the affected areas. It was discovered that bone cells seemed to cross the force-field, which eventually led in many cases to a union of the broken ends of bone.

Subsequent research has also focused on the use of electromagnetic forces to aid in the healing of inflammations.The theory is that every body cell contains a positive and a negative component. If all the positive and negative components are lined up properly, healing will occur more quickly. Some recent scientific studies appear to indicate positive results—for example, for some arthritic conditions.I played a minor role in one unscientific study, and met with varying results. I don't think we really understand enough about electromagnetic forces to make any definitive statements about their healing properties. If you want to try electromagnetic therapy on your arthritic foot or knee, discuss the possibilities with a podiatrist, orthopedic specialist, or other medical practitioner who may be familiar with the technique.

**Q.** Ultrasound therapy seems to be used for a variety of foot and leg maladies. I know how it is used as a diagnostic tool. But how do the sound waves help heal sore feet and legs? Do other, newer forms of physiotherapy work as well or better?

**A.** As ultrasound waves pass through body tissues they are turned into heat, which increases circulation.We know that increased circulation to a traumatized part of the body helps reduce inflammation more quickly. Therefore, when you are treated with ultrasound you are merely speeding up the healing process. The one time we definitely avoid ultrasound therapy is in treating a fracture. It appears to interfere with the natural healing process of broken bones. That is one reason why, for example, it is vital to determine whether a painful area around the sesamoid bone is the result of a fracture or an inflammation.

Ultrasound therapy has been used for quite a while, with varying degrees of success. There are now a few new modalities for physiotherapists to use, and laser therapy is one of them. Certain laser beams, which convert to heat once inside the body, seem to exhibit anti-inflammatory properties. Perhaps they will prove to be more successful in treating inflammations of the feet than their cousins were in removing plantar warts and ingrown toenails.

Last summer I discovered that a professional sports team was using a newer form of therapy known as diapulse/myopulse. When I asked the trainer about it he said he didn't know how it worked, but his injured players were certainly responding more positively than with other forms of anti-inflammatory treatment. Intrigued by the pulsating news, I set out to learn more about this novel form of physiotherapy.

Let me briefly summarize how diapulse/myopulse therapy works. The apparatus sends two different pulses through the injured area. These pulses seem to reduce inflammation more rapidly and effectively than other types of physiotherapy if used immediately after an injury occurs. However, the beneficial effects of diapulse/myopulse therapy diminish with time. It does not appear to be overly successful when used a few days or weeks after an injury. Therefore, its use at present appears to be limited to the treatment of those people who have almost

immediate access to it after being hurt.Those most likely
to benefit from it are athletes whose injuries are diagnosed
and aggressively and quickly treated.

**Q.** I was told that many of my aches and pains are due
to my having one leg longer than the other. I also know
that one of my feet is longer than the other. How can I
overcome this problem if it really is causing my discomfort?

**A.** According to Dr. Hamilton Hall, the orthopedic surgeon,
a half-inch (1 cm) discrepancy in the size of a person's
legs is within normal range.Anything less than that
difference cannot be blamed for all of a person's foot, leg,
knee, hip, and back problems, as some medical
professionals occasionally do.

Many types of medical professionals—and perhaps
even your tailor—are adept at accurately measuring the
length of your legs. If you think that you may have one leg
longer than the other, I suggest that you have a physician,
podiatrist, orthopod, chiropractor, or physiotherapist take
the measurements. If the difference is half an inch or less,
your problem probably lies elsewhere.If one leg is more
than 1 inch (2.5 cm) longer than the other, you should try
a 1/4-inch (6 mm) heel pad in the shorter leg for about one
month. If that doesn't work, you should be further evaluated
by a medical specialist to ascertain the next course of
action.

It is not unusual for one foot to be larger than the other,
unless the difference can be measured in inches rather
than in fractions of an inch. Aside from the trouble in
finding shoes that fit both feet properly, there is no major
problem with a small difference in size. Athletic shoes can

often be adjusted, using the laces, to fit both feet adequately. Dress and other types of shoes should be flexible enough to stretch to accommodate the larger foot. In cases where one foot is substantially larger than the other, the individual may have to purchase custom-made footwear—not an easy commodity to find these days.

**Q.** Is it true that most shoe stores have carpeted floors so that you won't be able to tell how little cushioning or support there is in their footwear?

**A.** No. Most shoe stores have carpeted floors to prevent the shoes you are trying on—and probably won't buy— from becoming worn or soiled. Incidentally, good athletic shoe stores will have five or six surfaces approximating those on which you play or exercise. For example, there will be a patch of wood flooring for basketball players, synthetic asphalt or turf surfaces for those who run or play baseball, soccer, football, and so on. By providing you with these different types of surfaces, the stores are helping you select the shoe that is right for your activity and feet.

**Q.** I am a ballet dancer. Like most people in my profession I have terrible feet. Is there anything I can do to prevent the host of foot problems that plague me and my fellow dancers?

**A.** Precious little. Probably 90 per cent of all ballet dancers have foot problems because of the abnormal positions of their toes when they dance. The tips of the toes were not designed to bear the excess amount of weight and stress to which they are often subjected. The worst position is when a dancer is spinning around or hopping up and down on "point." Eventually the muscles and tendons in the toes tighten dramatically and begin to contract. The result is hammer or mallet toes (the latter condition involves the joint between the first and second bones in the toe, rather than the second and third bones) and corns atop the toes. Also, it is quite common for ballet dancers to develop bunions because of the tremendous stress on the inside of the forefoot. I have seen numerous other problems in ballet dancers over the years, from damaged toenail beds, which leave their victims with a wide assortment of nail colors and shapes, to stress fractures. Last summer I treated one ballerina for plantar fasciitis, which was severe enough to force her to cancel some engagements. These are the prices you must pay if you constantly try to perform certain activities for which the human foot was not designed.

A word of advice is in order for parents of youngsters who want to take up ballet dancing. Children in their pre-teen years should not be allowed to do point work, because the bones in their feet are very vulnerable to damage while they are still growing. Moreover, their leg and foot muscles are usually not strong enough to support them in this awkward position, so they could hurt themselves when they try to get up on their toes. It would be wise to check out the instructors and the programs they follow to ascertain if their approach is in the best interests of your child.

**Q.** I was told by a podiatrist that I needed bunion surgery, which he said he could perform. My family doctor warned me that only an orthopedic surgeon is qualified to carry out such an operation. Whom do I believe?

**A.** This is not an easy question to answer. Both podiatrists and orthopedic surgeons are trained to perform bunion surgery. As I mentioned in Chapter Three, there are those in both professions who specialize in the "open" technique, those who use the "closed" method, and those who are adept at both procedures and determine which one to use based on the complexity of the case. In the U.S., most states allow podiatrists to do foot surgery. In Canada, each province has a different set of rules. If your province allows podiatrists to perform bunion surgery, you should be confident of his or her abilities as long as he or she is a certified D.P.M. (Doctor of Podiatric Medicine). In other parts of the world, particularly in Europe, chiropody schools are now allowed to teach foot surgery to their students. When it comes to bunion surgery, the operative word is confidence. Since both qualified podiatrists and orthopedic surgeons have been trained to perform bunion surgery, I would choose the doctor in whom I had the most confidence.

**Q.** I recently read that bunions can be operated on painlessly. Is this true? If so, who does such surgery?

**A.** All surgery today is basically painless. This is because either local or general anesthetics are administered to the patient before the operation. So, what we are talking about here is post-operative pain, which is now controlled much better than before for three reasons.

Firstly, surgery techniques have improved tremendously.

This means that there is significantly less trauma to the area being operated on. Secondly, the anesthetics administered for bunion surgery are longer acting, so that much of the immediate post-op pain is diminished. Thirdly, pain-killing medications are much more effective. As a result, long-term discomfort is minimized.

As I discussed in Chapter Three, there has been a lot of publicity about laser and minimal-incision surgery techniques to remove bunions.But regardless of the technique used, soft tissue is still being traumatized, and bone is being cut or shaved. All of this produces significant swelling and some discomfort. Moreover, complications, such as infections, can arise during the healing process. Therefore, bunion surgery is not to be taken lightly, even with advanced surgical techniques.The patient must understand that there will be some post-op discomfort, and will have to take the proper precautions to prevent any unpleasant side effects. A detailed discussion with the surgeon is in order before the decision is made to proceed with the operation.

**Q.** I think my two-year-old is toeing in excessively when she walks. Should I have her examined by a specialist now, or wait another year or so? My family doctor does not think it warrants attention at this point.

**A.** My feeling is that children who do not toe in or out excessively should be left alone if they are under the age of four. If your family doctor believes that the degree of abnormality is not serious, and if you have confidence in him or her, I would take that advice. If you are unsure, by all means seek a second opinion from a podiatrist or pediatric orthopod. You should also consult them if your child continues to toe in or out with no appreciable change after the age of four.

Should your child be diagnosed at birth or later as having a foot or lower leg abnormality, there are numerous non-invasive ways of correcting the fault with appliances designed to straighten the offending feet. As I mentioned in Chapter Three, recent advances in these appliances have made them much more effective and comfortable for the child to wear.

**Q.** I have heard about Morton's neuroma and neuromas between other toes. Can a person develop a neuroma elsewhere on the foot? I have had a sore spot on the side of one big toe for over a year, and my doctor cannot find the cause. Can you also tell me why the condition is called a neuroma? I thought a neuroma was a tumor.

**A.** The last shall be first here. Strictly speaking, a neuroma is a tumor. However, when we talk in this book about a neuroma of a nerve, we are referring to a swelling or inflammation of the nerve and the area around it. We are not discussing malignancies.

A neuroma can occur anywhere there is a nerve—in other words, throughout the body. The offended nerve is being pinched or impinged for a number of reasons. It is not uncommon for a tight shoe to result in an impinged nerve in the foot. Aside from between the toes, the most common neuroma in the foot is under a metatarsal head, particularly the first. It is also possible to develop a similar inflammation on the side of the big toe, so you may well have a neuroma. You will help your doctor make the diagnosis if you can describe your symptoms as a burning, tingling, numbing, and/or pins-and-needles sensation.

**Q.** You discuss in detail how certain exercises can harm the feet. Are there any types of exercises that are particularly good for the feet?

**A.** Walking, walking, and more walking! Naturally, you must be able to walk normally to benefit from this advice. If you are, there is no better exercise for your feet. Some people believe that rolling on soft-drink bottles or rolling pins will help strengthen the muscles in the feet; others think that foot massages will keep their feet fit. Well, whatever turns you on. The fact is that the muscles in your feet do not require special exercises to keep them fit. All they require is the opportunity to walk regularly in a biomechanically sound manner.

**Q.** I was told that the straighter the last of the shoe, the better it was for a person who over-pronated. Is it not true then that a perfectly straight-lasted shoe would totally eliminate over-pronation, without the need for orthotics?

**A.** No. Some athletic shoes are constructed so that they can control some of the excess rolling of the foot, which is over-pronation. However, no shoe of any type can totally prevent over-pronation. Therefore, a person with a severe pronation problem will still require orthotics, regardless of the type of shoes worn. People who have a rigid, slightly curved foot with a higher than normal arch will usually be more comfortable in a shoe with a curved last, since they will have a tendency to over-supinate rather than over-pronate. The curved last will help prevent them from rolling too much to the inside of the foot. If you are uncertain which shoe is best for you, take a good look at the shape of the shoe and seek the advice of a well-trained shoe salesperson.

**Q.** Are sandals—particularly those that have compartments for different toes—biomechanically sound?

**A.** If your feet are quite normal, and if you do not require the stability and shock absorption provided by athletic and some types of dress shoes, there is nothing wrong with wearing sandals, with or without compartments. However, if you do have a foot or lower leg abnormality, you would probably be much better off not wearing them. Besides, it would be rather difficult wearing the sandals with orthotics, particularly if the shoes have compartments. One of my patients tried wearing sandals three summers ago when it was so hot in Toronto. He gave up after one week of constant knee pain when he walked in them. So, you be the judge. If you are comfortable in sandals and do not suffer any lower limb or low back discomfort while wearing them, enjoy the cool breezes on your feet. One word of advice—don't wear them too long for the first couple of weeks. It takes a while for the feet to adjust to them.

**Q.** My feet are just plain tired at the end of the day. Does this mean that I have a biomechanical problem, or some systemic disorder? Or is this a natural occurrence after a long, hard day at work?

**A.** Tired feet is a very vague symptom. I would look first for a biomechanical problem, because tired feet can be like tired eyes—an indication that a correction is required. Biomechanical abnormalities often develop gradually, just like near- and far-sightedness. Perhaps your footwear is not providing you with sufficient support. If so, you may just need shoes that have more stability and shock absorption. If your biomechanics and footwear are deemed not to be the cause of your fatigued feet, the next step would be a complete physical examination to determine whether you have a systemic disorder. Should all the tests be negative or inconclusive, you might consider taking a relaxing holiday to rejuvenate yourself. Tired feet may be nothing more than a symptom of an over-worked, over-stressed individual.

**Q.** I see so many products on the market for foot care— athlete's foot remedies, corn pads and plasters, wart removers, odor-reducers and powders, and inserts that claim to cure or prevent all sorts of miseries. How can I know which ones will work effectively?

**A.** Let the buyer beware! I would not trust any over-the-counter or mail-order foot care product until I had had my feet properly examined by a medical specialist. If your doctor recommends a certain readily available product, by all means try it. However, it is quite easy for a layperson to misdiagnose a foot problem—for example, by confusing calluses and corns with warts. Therefore, you may purchase the right product for the wrong condition. I am particularly concerned about acid-based corn and callus pads, which can cause foot ulcers and infections if abused. I am also dubious of claims made by the manufacturers of inserts that are advertised as being able to effectively treat all types of problems. As I have explained throughout this book, your biomechanical abnormalities are unique and, if pronounced, require orthotics designed specifically for your feet.

**Q.** I tried to get into shape to compete in a triathlon, but always ran into injury roadblocks—my feet, my knees, my hips, and my lower back. Will I ever be able to realize my dream? You claim that triathlons are not as hard on the body as straight running.

**A.** Let me tell you about one of my patients who managed to compete almost pain-free in an Ironman triathlon, despite a series of nagging overuse injuries that continuously put him out of training. After you read his story you can decide for yourself if you want to achieve your goal.

Andrew undertook a running program without an understanding of what constitutes safe exercising. Andrew had been a part-time cyclist, but in 1985 he decided that he wanted to be fit faster. So he bought a pair of running shoes and began jogging, totally unaware that he had foot problems. He also made the mistake of running too far, too soon, and quickly developed a classic overuse syndrome, plantar fasciitis. His feet were so sore in the morning when he got out of bed that he had to rub them for fifteen minutes before he could walk.

Andrew went to his doctor, who accurately diagnosed his condition but failed to advise the proper course of action. Andrew was told to apply ice to the inflamed area (that part was fine) and to roll tennis balls under his feet. The pain abated, but only slightly. A friend suggested that he see a podiatrist, who recommended orthotics, which he purchased and received several weeks later. He described them as "large, heavy, and initially very uncomfortable." Moreover, they fit in his running shoes only, so he could not wear them most of the time. The plantar fasciitis disappeared; however, he soon developed severe leg cramps. The orthotics were adjusted several times, but the cramps persisted and he eventually discarded them.

Another friend suggested that Andrew see me. I suggested that he try a new lightweight pair of orthotics, and he agreed. As soon as he began wearing them the pain in his legs diminished and he had no further episodes of plantar fasciitis. He then began to pursue a dream of his— to compete in a triathlon—a 1.5 km swim, 40 km cycle, and a 10 km run.

Unfortunately, Andrew came down with a series of nagging injuries while training for his first triathlon, the most serious of which was an ilio-tibial band friction syndrome. He ignored the symptoms at first, but took notice when the pain became acute. His family doctor suggested that he pay a return visit to me, and I discovered that his orthotics had broken down somewhat from his heavy training program. I repaired the orthotics, and his discomfort subsided gradually, with the help of ice and stretching exercises. In the next few months he returned to my office for further orthotic adjustments and treatment for a host of new problems—muscle pulls, stiff toe joints on both feet, a broken baby toe, and anterior compartment pain. However, he was determined to continue training, and he managed to run two marathons in 1989 as well as compete in the challenging Ironman Triathlon in Hawaii. During this time he understood that the orthotics would not prevent his injuries, considering his extremely strenuous training program, but they helped him, he says, "ease the pain and resume running at my usual intensity." He claimed that he competed in the triathlon "virtually pain-free." Since then he has continued to run, although "at a lesser rate," and he continues to wear orthotics in his running shoes. I see him occasionally when he returns for adjustments to his orthotics.

Andrew is typical of the person who is determined to achieve a goal despite physical discomfort. He was quite willing to put up with a host of overuse injuries so he could compete in the triathlon, and ran close to 50 miles (80 km) a week, when not incapacitated, while in serious training. There is no doubt in my mind that he would have been unable to undertake such strenuous activity without the help of orthotics. Now that he has proved a point to himself, I hope he will reduce the risk of further overuse injuries, which may result in some long-term problems, and consider a less-stressful exercise regimen.

**Q.** My feet hurt all over when I get out of bed in the morning. Is this plantar fasciitis, even if the pain is more widespread?

**A.** Plantar fasciitis occurs only on the sole and heel of the foot. It can cause pain along the entire length of the plantar fasciae and where these ligaments attach to the heel bone in the rearfoot and the five metatarsal bones. If your pain is more widespread, you should have a complete physical examination. Your discomfort may be due to a number of conditions, from various types of arthritis to circulatory dysfunction to muscle contractions.

**Q.** If I have a biomechanical problem will I automatically eventually get some sort of foot disorder unless I begin wearing orthotics from now on for the rest of my life? On the other side of the coin, is the reverse also true—that is, can I suffer from foot disorders even if I have normal biomechanics?

**A.** Many people have biomechanical abnormalities but never suffer any discomfort whatsoever. If you over-pronate or over-supinate mildly and do not suffer from any physical deformity, there is no need for you to wear orthotics unless your doctor or podiatrist believes that you will develop serious problems later. This advice does not apply to children. If your child is diagnosed as having a foot or leg problem that will eventually lead to bone and joint and soft tissue disorders, you should have that child treated quickly to avoid subsequent trouble.

Abnormal biomechanics are not the only causes of foot problems. Poorly fitting shoes can also cause a wide variety of ailments, from corns to Achilles tendinitis.And, of course, many maladies, such as plantar warts and circulatory dysfunctions, result from systemic disorders.

**Q.** I recently read that stretching exercises don't really do much good. I run about 25 miles (40 km) a week and follow a comprehensive stretching exercise program. Yet I still have leg problems. Should I forget about stretching?

**A.** First of all, any athlete with leg problems should be examined by an expert in sports medicine. The trouble could be caused by any number of things, from improper warm-up techniques, poor biomechanics, circulatory disorders, and improperly fitting shoes, to muscle injuries.

As for stretching exercises, there has been some controversy over the past few years as to whether they benefit athletes. Stretching has been generally considered as one step in preparing the cardiovascular and pulmonary systems, and the muscles, for more intense activity. My discussions with athletes, including many baseball players, lead me to believe strongly that stretching exercises are definitely beneficial. However, if you believe that you can survive your workouts nicely without stretching, more power to you.

**Q.** I was told by my doctor that my hip pain was caused by an ilio-tibial band problem. Where is this band and why is it bothering my hip?

**A.** The ilio-tibial band is muscle tissue that runs from the hip joint down the outside of the leg and attaches at the head of the fibula. If the band has become over-stretched, which can happen for a number of reasons, including abnormal biomechanics in the foot and leg, it can become irritated at the hip joint or when it contacts the outside of the knee. The inflammation can be treated with a proper physiotherapy program and, if necessary, with orthotics to correct a biomechanical fault.

Seven years ago I treated a young woman who had just taken up running and who had begun experiencing severe pain on the outside of her left knee. She had initially thought that the pain was normal for a new runner and that it would gradually disappear. However, it gradually worsened to the point where it hurt even when she was walking.

I watched Sandy walk for a few minutes, and concluded that her problems were caused by over-pronation. I convinced her to invest in orthotics and had her undergo physiotherapy treatment—ice, ultrasound, and massages. She quickly recovered, and I saw her only once after that, about a year later when she switched to new, lighter orthotics.

A few months ago Sandy began to experience acute pain in her right hip. She had been running sporadically, and was often "overdoing it" when she got out on the track. She saw a specialist, who told her that the pain was caused by friction where the ilio-tibial band attaches beside the hip joint. She was given some exercises to do, which helped but did not solve her problems. She then decided to pay me a visit.

Sandy's orthotics had completely worn down. I suggested that she immediately buy a new pair, which she did, and her hip pain quickly disappeared. She is now running again without any problems.

The ilio-tibial band friction syndrome can be confused with other sports-related injuries. Therefore, if you suspect that your symptoms are similar to those described above you should be examined and treated by medical practitioners well versed in sports medicine.

**Q.** I recently lost a toenail in an accident. Is there anything I can do to ensure that it grows back properly?

**A.** It is very common after a toenail injury for the nail to fall off. It will normally grow back within twelve to eighteen months, about double the time for a fingernail, because of poorer circulation in the feet than in the hands.

Two things can go wrong after a toenail has been injured. Firstly, the nail-growing cells may be damaged in the accident and will never again produce a normal nail. Therefore, the new nail may grow misshapen. Nothing can be done to prevent this from occurring. If the new nail causes a lot of discomfort, some or all of it may have to be removed and the nail-growing cells destroyed. Fortunately, people can survive quite nicely without their toenails.

Secondly, the new nail may grow in with a fungal infection because the fungus found a moist, dark, warm breeding area in which to establish a toe-hold while the area was healing. Therefore, I recommend that the affected toe be treated regularly with an anti-fungal cream until the new nail has completely regrown—that is, for twelve to eighteen months.

**Q.** I lost my right foot in an industrial accident a few months ago. I am now learning to walk again with a prosthetic limb. Unfortunately, my left leg and foot have begun hurting me. Will I ever be able to walk comfortably again?

**A.** You will have to be patient. Tremendous strides have been made in the past few years in the development of lighter, more biomechanically sound prosthetics. However, it takes a lengthy period of healing, physiotherapy, and learning how to walk with an artificial limb before the body fully adjusts to the new situation. Eventually the hips, pelvis, and upper legs learn how to compensate for the loss of a lower leg and foot, and the biomechanics of walking normalize. You should be able to walk normally again; it just takes time.

**Q.** You have said that foot abnormalities can cause back aches. My chiropractor recently prescribed orthotics for my feet, because I had constant low back pain. My discomfort has eased, but I am still skeptical about the relationship. Is there any proof to back up this theory?

**A.** At this point my belief that certain low back problems can be attributed to foot dysfunctions is empirical. I have had many patients experience relief from back, hip, and knee pain with a correction of their biomechanical abnormalities. At present I am involved in a study with Dr. Hamilton Hall and the Canadian Back Institute that will examine data from computer gait analyses. We are trying to ascertain if there is a link between specific gait abnormalities and certain types of low back problems. As I write this book there is no way conclusively to prove such a relationship. But stay tuned!

I want to stress that not all low back disorders can be either directly or indirectly related to foot problems. There are far too many other factors involved that can have a profound effect on the functioning of the lower back.

**Q.** It seems that whenever I buy new ski equipment the sales personnel try to sell me skithotics. Why should I buy them if I have normal feet? Will they improve my skiing ability?

**A.** When you are skiing downhill the skithotics will hold the foot in a fairly neutral position—that is, they will prevent the foot from tilting to the inside or the outside, thereby improving your skiing mechanics. The skithotics will take a lot of the pressure off the knees when you are on a slalom course. When the feet are allowed to tilt or cave in, the knees will be forced much farther out to keep the skis neutral. This makes edging much more difficult when you are cutting from one side to the other at high speed. If you are skiing competitively, you will save precious fractions of seconds on your downhill run if you wear skithotics. Moreover, you will probably save your knees from unusual wear and tear.

**Q.** Last year I had plantar fasciitis, which my doctor treated with a cortisone injection and inserts. Two months ago, after running a marathon, I developed severe Achilles tendinitis. My doctor refused to inject me with cortisone. Why?

**A.** The Achilles tendon is one of those areas of the body that reacts adversely to cortisone injections. It seems that the cortisone actually eats away at and weakens the Achilles tendon, and could eventually cause it to rupture. If this happens surgery will be required to repair the tendon, because of the poorer circulation to that part of the body, which impedes healing. If you have Achilles tendinitis and your doctor recommends a cortisone injection, I would get a second opinion.

Incidentally, it is not all that uncommon for someone with plantar fasciitis to subsequently dvelop Achilles tendinitis, or vice versa. This is because of the lever effect at the bottom of the ankle joint. When the plantar fasciae are being over-stretched, they try to "borrow" fibers from the Achilles tendon to eliminate the problem. This places undue stress on the Achilles tendon, which runs from the back of the calcaneus (heel bone) to the calf muscle. If the Achilles tendon is tight to begin with (as is the case with women who wear high-heel shoes regularly), it will become over-stretched and inflamed. This sets up the possibility of Achilles tendinitis. The opposite is also true, and Achilles tendinitis can eventually lead to plantar fasciitis.

**Q.** I am a seventy-three-year-old lady who still likes to take long walks regularly. My doctor advised me to get a good pair of orthopedic shoes, because my feet have begun to bother me. I've been to many stores, but the salespeople keep trying to sell me shoes that aren't "orthopedic." Why can't I find orthopedic shoes?

**A.** Because, according to Dr. Hamilton Hall, there is no such thing as an orthopedic shoe. After World War Two some types of oxford shoes included metatarsal supports and higher arches, and they became known as orthopedic shoes, though there was nothing particularly "orthopedic" about them. Today's walking/running shoes provide far greater stability, flexibility, and shock absorption than the oxfords. I would recommend that you buy one of the pairs of running shoes I discussed in Chapters Six and Eight.

One American shoe manufacturer, P.W. Minor, makes an "extra-depth" shoe, which is very deep to allow for the insertion of soft insoles that help alleviate irritation caused by the lining of shoes. One of their models can even be heated—for five to ten minutes with, for example, a hair dryer—to adapt to the shape of any foot no matter how deformed. This type of shoe would be perfect for geriatric feet that have often become misshapen through disease or neglect of a biomechanical fault, and particularly for those with large bunions.

**Q.** What is it like being the foot care consultant to the Toronto Blue Jays baseball team? Is treating professional athletes any different from caring for the general population?

**A.** I was fortunate in 1982 to be asked by Dr. Ron Taylor, a former major league pitcher, to examine a number of the Blue Jays players with foot problems. Dr. Taylor, the head of the S.C. Cooper Sports Medicine Clinic at Mount Sinai Hospital in Toronto, eventually asked me to be available as a consultant to the team, and I have been ever since. As with most professional teams, the trainer is the first line of defense when it comes to injuries. Tommy Craig, the Blue Jays' trainer, will then discuss the case with Dr. Taylor, who will evaluate the injury and decide what course of action to take. Dr. Taylor will also decide if the player should be examined by any other specialist. In my particular case, there is an overlap between Dr. Alan Gross, the team's orthopedic surgeon, and myself. The three of us will often discuss a specific case together before a decision is made concerning one of the players.

The major difference in treating a professional athlete as opposed to the general public is the pressure to get the player back in action as quickly and safely as possible, particularly during the playing season. Yet in all my years in association with the Blue Jays, there has never been any pressure to put a player back on the field before he is ready. In fact, the Blue Jays prefer to allow the athlete to heal at his own pace, rather than take measures to speed up the natural healing process. It is not in the best interests of either the player or the team to jeopardize a career for the sake of trying to win a few extra games. On the other hand, professional athletes want to get back on the field as soon as possible, so they are usually very co-operative patients when it comes to following the recommendations and instructions of the trainers and doctors. Also, most players realize that their livelihood depends on taking care of themselves, and are in far better shape than the general public. As a result they tend to heal much faster and suffer fewer injuries than most other people in proportion to the amount of activities performed.

Many of the Blue Jays players I examine have problems similar to those mentioned throughout this book. The treatments they receive are also quite similar to those outlined in the book. The positive response of the players and the rest of the organization has made my nine years with the team a highlight of my professional career, and I thank them for giving me the opportunity to work with such an outstanding group of individuals.

**Q.** Why would anybody want to become a podiatrist?

**A.** I am often asked this question. I really enjoy examining feet; in fact, they are often a fascinating road map of a person's life. In all seriousness, podiatry is a very rewarding field. About eight in ten people will eventually suffer from foot discomforts of one type or another, and most of them can be treated quickly, efficiently, and effectively.

Sometimes, relief from pain is almost immediate, and what more could a doctor wish than to effect a speedy recovery? Also, podiatry is very much where the action is—sports medicine, of which foot care is a major component, is an exploding field, and as the population ages, geriatric medicine is also growing rapidly. The majority of my patients are athletically active or senior citizens or both.  So, as long as I practice podiatry, I will never be bored or out of work!

# Index